BODYSCULPTING *for* BOMBSHELLS

Fast and Easy Fitness for Loving Your Body and Feeling Desirable

Vivi Stutz

Book Interior and layout Design by Quest Publications
Email: questpublications@outlook.com
Website: www.questpub.questforgod.org

ACKNOWLEDGMENTS

Many thanks to my art department!

Thank you to Rosa Sophia for editing this book. Her website can be viewed at: www.rosasophia.com.

Thank you to Karin Mansson for hair and make up during the photo shoot.

Thank you to Tony Abruzzo for beta-reading, editing and being a patron of the arts.

CONTENTS

PART 4: CREATING BEAUTY: ADVANCED EXERCISE TECHNIQUES AND THE ART OF BODYSCULPTING .. 149

PART 1: THE BASICS

Chapter 1

EMBRACING BEAUTY:
THE BOMBSHELL PHILOSOPHY

There is a bombshell in every woman. It's our nature. Femininity, when it has the freedom to be expressed in its fullness, is forceful and gentle, assertive and yielding, sexual and nurturing at the same time. The feminine nature is multi-faceted in co-existing opposites, but we rarely materialize the expression of all aspects that live within us. We disown one part or another to conform to social norms within our respective cultures, and most frequently, we split off physical awareness and expression because we deem it unacceptable.

We are constantly at odds with our bodies.

Can you name one woman who is not at odds with her body? Maybe you can, but it's rare. Our body becomes a battlefield of expectations about who we think we should be and our own desire to be at peace with who we are. We fight endless battles of self-criticism and self-improvement, or we disconnect from awareness of our bodies altogether.

Resolving the dilemma is harder than it seems. We veer in and out of buying into social expectations, returning to body-awareness only when we feel good about ourselves. Sometimes we admit we have a body, sometimes we ignore it and act as if we don't.

You know your self-esteem shouldn't depend on how you look, but divorcing self-esteem from appearance only works for some women, not others. Some women are naturally beautiful, and others have rock-solid self-esteem despite the absence of what their society defines as physical beauty. Most of us are neither blessed with natural beauty nor rock-solid self-esteem, and most of us enjoy physical and sensual expression only on "good days".

Denying the unfairness of genes works only to some extent. In truth, nature isn't fair.

As a woman in the United States, how you appear at any given age is part of your currency. It's a non-monetary stock market investment. Men's value appreciates with age. Their portfolio and earning potential increases, and they're perceived as more desirable because of the increased security they provide. Women's value depreciates with age, because youth is associated with fertility and health. Even men who've had plenty of children with numerous ex-wives are attracted to women who suggest fertility and health. In other words, youth. It's wired into our evolutionary instinct.

Overweight women are perceived as "out of control," while overweight men are merely perceived as "lacking discipline." The road to eating disorders and Body Dysmorphic Disorder is already paved.

Women who reach the age of 35 are considered "past their prime." Desirability has an expiration date. Larger sized women are "not supposed to" feel desirable because the beauty ideal dictates clothing sizes fit for teenage girls.

It gets worse. A *TIME* magazine article from June 29, 2015 about the social pressures of receiving cosmetic procedures quoted a study that found above-average looking people earning up to $230,000 more throughout their life time than their average looking counterparts.

How do we withstand the pressure?

We either conform by entering the manic quest for perfection, or we split off sensual awareness of our bodies because the feelings of inadequacy are too painful. We sway back and forth between these extremes, liking ourselves most when we are closest to the expectation we hold. We rarely feel at home in our own skin.

If we want to become whole again, we must boldly claim ownership of our physical self. Unedited physical expression is sumptuous, exuberant, sensual and highly desirable if we suspend judgment and allow ourselves to be present in our bodies. A woman who owns her physical expression without shame is desirable at any size or age. Her innate sensuality defies cultural norms. She'll be a whole lot happier, too. She has recovered her *bombshell nature.*

How is it done? The first step is giving yourself permission. You too, are a bombshell at heart. The next step is getting back into your body through movement. Use exercise to enhance and heal the relationship you have with your body. Beauty is a mindset, not a clothing size.

When was the last time you felt truly comfortable in your body? It was most likely after you were physically active. Movement awakens body awareness.

Exercise can alter body size and shape if you desire to do so. If you are truly uncomfortable with your size and shape, change it. You can make your body a work of art and shape it like a sculpture. It takes time, effort and commitment, but it can be done.

However, exercising for the quest of perfection can be emotionally devastating and damage self-esteem. Don't exercise to find yet another way of beating yourself up. Define your own goals and make loving your body the highest priority. Treat your physical self like a temple that houses your spirit.

Exercise is on everyone's to-do list, yet there's always a good reason not to. For many people, exercise is annoying; it's not fun, and it gets boring. The process of fitness can be as daunting as fixing an engine if you don't know how it's done. Reading large volumes on exercise science isn't everyone's idea of a good time, and fitness magazines offer quick fixes that rarely yield results.

We don't need yet another failed attempt.

I've tried to keep this book short and sweet. Knowing a few simple facts about exercise reduces time commitment and frustration. The following pages won't give you a complicated workout regime but an understanding of what works and why. The practical instruction will be a sample whole body workout which you can use, alter, or build from. It's all you need to get started, get comfortable in your skin again, and see significant changes or lose weight if you wish. It's not rocket science, after all.

Don't wait until you lost weight, and don't beat yourself up if you haven't been able to. You can, but you don't need to change your body size to recover your bombshell nature. Larger women can sculpt their bodies into voluptuous shapes. *Sports Illustrated* of February 2016 featured Ashley Graham on the cover, a size 16 swimsuit model. When artfully sculpted, curvy is feminine beauty.

I credit my friend Amber Rice, a San Diego-based marriage and family therapist, with modeling ownership of beauty at any size. I learned from her that bombshells come in all sizes and ages, because beauty emerges from ownership.

CHAPTER 2

BUILDING BEAUTY: WHAT YOU NEED TO KNOW ABOUT EXERCISE

Exercise is annoying. If it wasn't, you'd be doing it. You'd be exercising regularly, you would look and feel fantastic, and you'd be so accustomed to receiving compliments about your great shape that it wouldn't be any more exciting than collecting the mail.

Maybe you'll argue that exercise isn't annoying because you feel great after you do it, but there's still something about your physical shape that's nagging you or you wouldn't read a book about it. Perhaps you exercise occasionally but don't stick with it for reasons you can't put your finger on.

Maybe you've put it off because you don't know how it's done, or you put in countless hours at the gym and it doesn't make the difference you anticipated. You feel stuck in a body you'd rather hide, and exercise is too time consuming. You think you're not cut out to look or feel good because you're too big-boned, too short or too old, or you don't have the right genes. You may even think you need to lose weight *before* you start exercising.

Learning to exercise correctly is surprisingly simple and can be summarized into short, easy-to-follow steps. It'll be far less annoying if you know what you're doing and why.

The strongest motivating factor for exercise is the ability to reap its many rewards. Often, people quit because they haven't learned how to do it correctly. Investments without returns are worth dropping, after all.

Once you experience the physical transformation of body composition—less fat, more lean mass, faster metabolism, higher energy levels, graceful mobility, comfortable flexibility, improved health and the joy of inhabiting a body you love—it becomes harder to quit. Why would you give something up that makes you feel better, more beautiful, and more energetic?

Investments that reap high returns are worth keeping.

Learning to exercise correctly is not as self-explanatory as it might seem. You must have had at least one friend who worked out for hours every day, limped home, complained about it and quit. They quit because the investment had no viable returns, so you wouldn't want to waste your time this way.

However, don't blame your genes or the gym. Who taught your friend how to implement exercise science? Was it a high school gym teacher, or did your friend read a stack of fitness magazines that promised results?

There is no single exercise that guarantees results. If there were, we wouldn't be battling our bodies; we'd be doing the right exercise and looking great.

All exercises work if you know how to:

A) Understand the different modes of exercises

B) Grow a muscle

C) Combine exercises

You need an owner's manual and a road map. Once you have the tools, you'll achieve the changes you were looking for. The ideal mixture of cardiovascular and weight training will speed up your metabolism, skyrocket your energy levels, change your body composition and improve your health. Your owner's manual is basic knowledge of exercise science, and your road map is The Basic Workout provided in the Practical Instruction section of this book.

COMBINE WEIGHT TRAINING, CARDIOVASCULAR EXERCISE, AND STRETCHING

This will take less time than you think, and you can play favorites when it comes to particular exercises as long as you don't discriminate. If you use only one mode of exercise, such as the treadmill, you are short-changing yourself and not getting the most out of what the gym has to offer.

Each type of exercise serves a different purpose. Cardiovascular training increases energy levels. Weight training builds muscle. Stretching keeps you flexible. If you've exercised at a gym before, have you utilized only one or two modes of exercise? If so, were you fully satisfied with the results?

If you specialize on spending hours on the treadmill, you'll have more energy and feel fit, but your body will stay soft and flabby. You'll get tight hamstrings or pain in your back. Your upper body will begin to lose the battle against gravity and you'll hunch forward, which will ruin your posture and only lead to more back pain.

If you favored lifting weights, you may be toned and shapely, but you'll wonder why you don't feel energetic. Your mobility will decrease as your movements become limited from tight muscles. Watch your step. Has it gotten shorter?

If you stretch like a cat, you'll be graceful and in less pain than the average person in your age group, but you'll never have straight lean lines of muscle mass. Gravity will get you when its pull becomes stronger than the pull of your muscles, and you'll hunch. You might feel fit, but you won't be. Try outrunning parking enforcement before they ticket your car. Gasping for air yet?

WHICH MODE OF EXERCISE SERVES WHICH PURPOSE?

Let's take a quick look at the purpose of each mode of exercise. This will be part of your owner's manual. We'll go through each mode in greater detail in the related chapters. For now, you need to know the basics.

Cardiovascular fitness relates to picking up speed and keeping it up. When we fantasize about fitness, we usually envision having the energy and endurance we once took for granted a decade or two ago.

Cardiovascular exercise is a low to medium intensity activity such as running on a treadmill or running outdoors, or using an elliptical walker or StairMaster. It's a mode of exercise you can sustain over long periods of time.

At a gym, the majority of women will spend their time on cardio equipment. The goal of hour-long cardiovascular training is burning fat. Yes, cardiovascular exercise burns calories and fat, but it will never burn fat as effectively as it will when it's combined with weight lifting. Also, cardiovascular training yields results according to heart rate training zones, which you must know if you don't want to waste your time. We'll cover the mystery of heart rate training zones in the chapter on cardiovascular exercise.

The main function of cardiovascular exercise is strengthening the heart and improving oxygen consumption. Improved oxygen consumption means that higher levels of oxygen circulate through your system and lung capacity is greater. Oxygen boosts your energy better than cocaine; it's legal and it won't destroy your dopamine receptors. Just kidding. Oxygen is a miracle drug. Try it.

Most health benefits are related to cardiovascular training. Type 2 Diabetes can be improved with a combination of exercise and nutrition. High blood pressure can be lowered—the systolic and diastolic pressure. Triglycerin, the level of fat in the blood, can be lowered. A stronger heart, obviously, is a protective factor against heart attacks.

At the gym, weight training is the less popular pastime—lifting heavy objects to build lean muscle mass and increase strength.

Why do you need strength? Even if your boyfriend/husband/secret lover carries your grocery bags and works on your car, you still need strength. Strength is a byproduct of straight, lean muscular lines across your body where flab once resided. You may not lift weights because you want to get stronger, but you do want lean muscle mass. Every cut, rip, or straight line on a toned body is muscle mass. We cannot tone fat, only muscle.

Lifting heavy objects burns an awful lot of calories. You can't burn as many calories in an hour on a treadmill as you can when lifting weights. Increased lean muscle mass burns more calories than the absence of muscle does, so building muscle mass can speed up a sluggish metabolism. The more lean muscle mass you have, the higher your metabolism.

Stretching is essential because it helps regain or maintain your range of motion. Range of motion is the angle at which your bones can move across a joint. If you don't stretch, you'll get tighter as you age. The range of motion becomes smaller until movement is very limited. Tight muscles pull on joints and bones, causing pain. The tighter a muscle is, the more prone you will be to pulls, injuries, and pinched nerves.

CARDIOVASCULAR EXERCISE AND WEIGHT LIFTING USE DIFFERENT ENERGY SYSTEMS

Feed a muscle, starve the fat. Know the difference.

To do so, you need to understand the body's energy systems. Energy systems are the metabolical processes that turn food into energy, which we refer to as calories. You need to know which system does what, so you can tailor your time investment to what you want to accomplish.

One (anaerobic) energy system utilizes stored sugars to do heavy work for very short periods of time. The next two (anaerobic) energy systems use sugars for heavy work that lasts half a minute or up to three minutes. The last (aerobic) energy system provides energy for light work that takes very long periods of time.

Anaerobic means the systems need sugars or calories as fuel. Aerobic means the system uses oxygen and eventually fat storages.

For example, lifting a heavy box is hard work for a short period of time. Carrying heavy grocery bags is hard work that takes a longer period of time. Running or fast walking is light work that may take a very long time. Each activity draws fuel from a different energy system.

Since running or fast walking both use the aerobic energy system that will turn to fat storages when sugars run out, cardiovascular training has become the most popular activity for weight loss. It works, but the downside is that you have to run several hours every day to see significant weight loss.

There's a more effective way to get the job done, which is why I cautioned you to combine all modes of exercise for best results. The trick is to use the right energy system at the right time.

Weight lifting burns far more calories than cardiovascular training, in far less time. Weight lifting will increase and maintain a higher metabolism over time. As noted earlier, muscle needs more calories to sustain itself.

Feed a muscle, starve the fat.

A muscle needs fuel to get work done. The fuel is calories, or more specifically, stored sugars.

You may claim you've had no sugar today, but your sneaky body has turned a lot of your food into glucose and stored it as glycogen. Glucose is a pretty word for sugar. Glucose is made from the simple or complex carbohydrates you ate. When carbohydrates are converted into glycogen and stored in blood, muscle, and various other locations, the sugar becomes fuel.

Feed the muscle by eating complex carbohydrates before lifting weights. You'll burn the calories during the workout, the muscles will be happy because they had enough fuel, and they'll grow during rest.

Weight lifting creates an afterburn, which means the metabolism kicked into high gear from doing heavy work. The afterburn lasts up to twelve hours. You'll burn more calories even while resting on the couch, which comes in handy for weight loss.

However, if you don't feed the muscle before doing heavy work, it gets messy. Heavy work needs heavy fuel. If you have no stored glucose in your system because you starved yourself, the body will begin to break down its own protein as fuel. Muscle and tissue are made from protein. Using up your own lean muscle mass as fuel is a bad idea, especially if your goal is to build muscle and increase metabolism.

You may have heard a lot of talk about eating protein before and after lifting weights. Yes, muscle needs extra protein for building, but it doesn't matter when you eat it. You can add protein to the carbohydrates as fuel before weight lifting, but protein isn't an ideal source for quick energy. Protein takes up to three hours to digest. Carbohydrates are available as fuel as quickly as thirty minutes after eating.

As long as you consume enough protein during the day, you're covered. We'll go over protein intake when we discuss nutrition.

Cardiovascular training is less capricious. You don't need to worry about feeding your muscles. During cardiovascular training, the muscles don't do heavy work; they do light work over long periods of time.

Cardiovascular training turns more easily to drawing from fat storages when fuel runs out. It's an evolutionary perk to guarantee survival. If you were a tribal hunter, you may need to migrate and hunt for a long time on an empty stomach before you catch your dinner. Or you may need to migrate until you find vegetarian food sources.

During cardiovascular training, you mimic migration. You keep moving for long periods of time. Running on nearly used up fuel is the right time to draw from fat storages. Evolution set it up that way. You have to be able to keep moving until you secure food supplies or the human species may die off.

Feed the muscle so it can grow. Take in calories when they are needed. Deplete fat storages by migrating on cardio equipment. Run on empty when you can afford to.

One way of maximizing returns is lifting weights first and using stored glucose. Follow this with cardiovascular exercise to deplete fat storages. You'll build muscle and lose fat.

There are additional ways of kicking a slow metabolism into high gear. Let's dedicate the next chapter to it.

INCREASING AND MAINTAINING METABOLISM IS KEY TO WEIGHT LOSS

Are you sick of struggling with your weight? Are you frustrated with diets? Diet and changing nutritional habits are important, but the bad guy in the game is a slow metabolism.

Increasing and maintaining a higher metabolic rate is essential for losing weight and keeping it off.

For the sake of clarity, metabolic rate means the rate at which your body burns calories. Your metabolism may be naturally slow or fast, depending on several genetic factors as well as habitual activity levels.

If you have a slow metabolism, your body is geared for survival. You'd be the lucky one who'd still be standing when a starvation period set in, let's say during the Stone Age. Unfortunately, we don't value outlasting starvation periods a whole lot in present day America, and you don't care much for your body's special talent.

If you have a high metabolism, you'll know. You're the one who could always eat what she wanted without gaining weight.

Unfortunately, both slow and fast metabolisms are subject to aging, and that's when things go haywire. After the age of thirty, the body begins to break down its lean muscle mass. It's the beginning of a steady decline. If you had a fast metabolism, you may not notice until your mid-thirties. After the mid-thirties, it'll get more dramatic with every decade.

Muscle mass requires more calories to sustain itself. Once muscle begins to disappear, your body's caloric needs decline. You may not eat more than you used to, but inexplicable weight gain sets in. Taking it off is harder than it used to be. With increasing age, we turn chubby.

Once you notice the inexplicable weight gain, your rational reaction may be to turn to dieting.

Dieting may be necessary if you have more than 15 pounds to lose, and I recommend enlisting a medically supervised diet program. If you must, get help from qualified professionals. Unsupervised diets can be harmful to your health.

Some medically supervised diets are so stringent that you may not be permitted to exercise, but this is only the case for severe obesity and only in the beginning stages.

In the absence of severe and medically critical obesity, diets are best combined with exercise. The reason is not losing weight faster, but increasing and maintaining metabolism.

Crash diets trigger the alarm system of starvation mode. Diets without exercise also trigger starvation mode, only less rapidly. When starvation mode sets in, your faithful body will do its best to save your life by slowing down its metabolic rate. Yes, thanks a lot. But bodies are geared toward survival, and we have to collaborate respectfully with this valuable function or we will end up hating the body that serves us so well.

Starvation mode is in effect when you notice the weight loss slowing down during dieting. You'll still reach your target weight if you're patient, but then you're faced with a dilemma.

The weight came off, but your metabolism is slower than ever. Perhaps you've even lost some muscle mass, decreasing metabolic needs further.

Either you stick with the low caloric intake your body now requires, or you'll regain the weight rapidly. If you used a supervised diet program, you may receive help tapering off the diet without regaining the weight, but few people are able to keep it off unless they exercise.

Luckily, your goals and your body's survival functions can all get along by negotiating your diet, your metabolism, and your target weight. Use diplomatic skill with your body and create win-win situations. Honor your body's survival instincts by avoiding starvation mode and work diligently at increasing and maintaining your metabolism.

How is it done? Pair a reasonable diet with a reasonable regimen of cardiovascular exercise and weight lifting. Build lean muscle mass. The more muscle you have, the more calories you need. If you keep building muscle while dieting, you increase your metabolic rate instead of slowing it down too much.

Don't wait until you lose the weight. Do it all at once. This will make it easier to keep the weight off once you have lost it.

Here's another handy fact about metabolism: bodies adapt and build habits.

The more you increase your metabolism through cardiovascular training and weight lifting, the more your body gets used to it. If you consistently spike up your metabolism, the body becomes accustomed to burning calories at a higher rate. It's called changing your metabolic baseline. Changing the metabolic baseline translates into changing the body's previous comfort zone of burning calories slowly to burning calories at a higher rate.

There's a catch, though.

Your body is accustomed to a set point of weight and will react a bit nervously when you intend to change it. Your body is also a tad inflexible when it comes to changing the metabolic baseline.

What do you do? Use diplomacy. Honor the fact that the body takes a while to get used to a new comfort zone and help it along with consistent practice.

A little bit of exercise daily is better than a lot of exercise twice a week. Thirty minutes a day can do a lot to change your metabolic baseline.

You may not be able to fit cardiovascular and weight training into a thirty-minute session, but you can spend half an hour on each, or alternate between weight lifting days and cardiovascular days. Or you can combine cardio and weights on some days, and fit in shorter cardiovascular sessions on alternate days.

Long hours at the gym are counter-productive. Committing to that much time is rarely sustainable. Unless you seriously want to spend long hours at the gym every day, it will be more productive to exercise for shorter periods of time.

Cardiovascular exercise can be done every day, even though you should take a minimum of one day off for rest. If you're running, you shouldn't run more than 30 miles per week because of the impact on the knees. If you are using cardiovascular equipment of low impact (such as an elliptical walker or bicycle) you can exceed 30 miles.

Weight lifting cannot be done every day. Beginners must work the entire body including all nine major muscle groups two to three times a week, allowing for a 48-hour resting period. Lift weights every other day.

Split routines will be discussed in greater detail in another chapter. You can split upper and lower body weight training into alternate days to cut down the time commitment, but you would need to head to the gym six days a week. Six days a week is a lofty commitment, and also less sustainable.

Shoot for weight training three times a week if you can, and fill in with shorter cardiovascular sessions as often as you can stand it.

Don't forget stretching. Stretch 10 to 15 minutes after every bout of exercise.

Both cardio and weights will spike your metabolism if the intensity is high enough. We'll cover intensity for both modes of exercise in separate chapters. First, let's do away with the myth of bulky women.

MUSCLE DOES NOT BECOME BULKY ON WOMEN

If you want to see one hell of a difference, you may need to lift heavier weights than you think.

In case you're concerned, lean muscle mass on women creates the lean, toned look—not the bulky one. That is, unless you have an unusually high amount of testosterone running through your system, which is rare. You'd already know if you had high levels of male hormones, because you'd have several issues that come with hormonal imbalance. Are you a woman sporting a beard? Do you have a deep, raspy voice and a large Adam's apple? No? Then you're fine. You won't get bulky.

Even for male or female bodybuilders, building bulk requires nearly superhuman effort along with dedication, discipline, sacrifice, highly specialized training and sports nutrition. If getting bulky was as easy as lifting a heavy dumbbell or two, all men would look like superheroes. They don't, do they? It's not easy and it doesn't happen by accident. Bulky physiques are rare, for a good reason.

Muscle is anything that's firm on your body. Any line, rip or curve is muscle. We all want firm lines, but we're afraid the firm lines would turn into pumpkin-sized clobbers.

Here's a personal trainer joke. A new client comes in and says, "I want to get toned, but I don't want any muscle."

The trainer replies, "What are we going to tone? Your fat?"

It can't be done. If you want the firm lines, you have to build muscle.

Muscles need to receive enough stimulus to grow, which means you need to move from light to heavy weights to provide the necessary stimulus for growth. Heavy is subjective, but we will cover gauging the right amount of weight for you in the chapter on weight training.

If you're still on the fence about the dangers of getting bulky, I dare you to run an experiment.

Go ahead and build up to lifting "heavy." Build up slowly and safely, and see what happens. See if you like it. At worst, you'll look like Madonna. If you don't like her, no problem. Losing muscle is easier than gaining it. Lighten the weights and the muscles will get smaller. Or, if you passionately hate your muscled look, take a two- to four-week hiatus from weight lifting.

Muscle develops only as a response to demand. If there is no more demand, it will atrophy. Atrophy means the muscle shrinks, so it'll disappear in no time if you don't like it.

Like it and keep it, or dislike it and lose it. You'll learn a lot about bodysculpting by experimenting with muscle sizes. You can make muscle bigger or smaller and change looks as often as you like. Treat it like a theme party. Be Madonna for one party and Gwyneth Paltrow for another.

A fine perk of heavy lifting is that you can burn 700 calories or more in an hour. Heavy lifting is followed by a massive afterburn. In my mind, the afterburn following heavy weight lifting makes it feel as if fat is rapidly melting off my frame.

Let's bust another myth. Muscle fiber doesn't turn into fat tissue when you quit weight training. Muscle fiber and fat tissue are different materials. Muscle is built from strands of protein. Fat is adipose tissue. One cannot convert into the other.

If you lose body fat, the fat cells deflate. You can't lose fat cells; they'll stay where they are. The mean little things are constantly on call. Fat cells will inflate again if excess calories need to be stored. The location of your fat cells is genetically determined.

The location of muscle fiber and its type is also genetically determined. There are different types of muscle fiber. There's one for strength, one for a mixture of strength and endurance, and one for endurance only.

Men have a genetically higher distribution of strength fiber in their upper bodies. It's easier for men to build large upper body muscle based on their fiber type. Men's lung capacity is also greater. Women have far less strength fiber distribution in their upper bodies, but almost the same amount of strength fiber in their legs. Theoretically, you could build rather large leg muscles.

I recommend watching the weight load on the leg muscles so you get the exact size you want. We typically want our legs slim but muscular. Think of female cyclists. The outer portion of their thighs, called the *vastus lateralis*, can become massive from excessive training. If leg muscles become larger than you like, decrease the weights.

Female upper bodies thrive on heavy weights. You can't go too heavy on the triceps, located on the backside of your upper arm. Fighting flab requires heavy lifting. Shoulders will turn into a beautifully rounded cut. Bicep muscles will complement the straight lean line of well-defined triceps.

I've talked countless female clients into lifting heavier than they'd planned, and I haven't come across a single woman who didn't like her new arms.

Be aware of the in-between period when you're changing body composition, and don't mistake it as growing bulk. As a reminder, changing body composition means increasing lean muscle mass and decreasing fat tissue. When you first begin increasing muscle, it can look as if you're getting bigger. There are still layers of fat on top of the newly developing muscle. Don't worry; it's a transition. Once you lose fat, the straight lean lines will emerge. Muscle tissue is denser than adipose tissue, and your overall size will become smaller.

If achieving a smaller size is not your goal, you may be satisfied with the merits of the in-between period. Building muscle underneath fat tissue will tighten your figure into luscious curves. A previously flabby stomach can be firm and shapely in its fullness. A full-figured waist can turn into a glorious hourglass. Large buttocks can be lifted and tightened. Think Jennifer Lopez. Would we advise her to be stick-thin? Size can be an advantage if beautifully sculpted.

If in doubt about your work of art, ask for a man's opinion. He'll tell you whether you've succeeded in sculpting the extra pounds into the physique of a Greek goddess.

Here's another perk of heavy lifting which I adore. Theoretically, you can't get rid of cellulite. I haven't found anything in the professional literature that suggests you can. Yet, I've seen cellulite disappear on clients and myself. As cellulite-ridden as I was in my twenties, there's nothing left of it in my mid-forties. I've seen it on hundreds of female clients who dared to build muscular thighs, hips, and buttocks. It may be that fat cells deflate with weight loss and the skin tightens when it expands across muscular lines. I can't back it up scientifically, but I know it works. You can look far better in a bikini in your fifties than in your twenties if you build muscle.

Are you up for the experiment of heavy lifting? I'll assume you are. How could you resist? Remember to build slowly from light to heavy, and don't get carried away by the enthusiasm of getting started.

"NO PAIN, NO GAIN" RAN OUT OF FASHION IN THE 1980s

Don't brag about getting sore. It's no reason to be proud.

You've heard it before, I'm sure: "I went to the gym, and I'm so sore! I worked out!"

It's a popular battle cry at any gym, but from a professional point of view, it's advertising that you don't know what you're doing. And worse, you've caused yourself an injury and now you're so proud of it that you tell everyone: "I went to the gym yesterday and I worked very hard on ruining my shoulder joints, knees, or elbows. I did great! I'm only about 20 years away from giving myself arthritis. I did well today. I got something done!"

"No pain, no gain" is another myth about exercise, originating in the 1980s. It's not only outdated, it's soon to be ancient.

How do you know you're sore?

The perception of soreness is highly subjective. One client may feel sore after lifting a three-pound dumbbell. Another client denies feeling sore after tearing up his muscles and being unable to lift his arm.

Let's identify a *right* and a *wrong* kind of soreness.

The *right* kind of soreness announces its presence 36 hours post workout. I call it the muscles' awakening, caused by increased blood flow and oxygen transport. You'll feel minor tightness, heaviness, fatigue or tenderness. Growing a muscle requires straining it just past its previous capacity, so there is a microscopic injury. A microscopic injury is appropriate. Increased blood flow is part of the healing process. The muscles will look bigger or "pumped" temporarily due to minor swelling. The sensation should be noticeable but pleasant. You should notice that you did work, but you should never be in pain.

The *wrong* kind of soreness is pain. The muscles are not microscopically but majorly injured, and become so stiff and painful you can barely move. Repeated major injury to the muscle tissue leads to arthritis. In the worst case scenario, muscle can tear and if incorrectly rehabilitated, grow back mildly deformed.

You can get painfully sore from weight lifting or from running 20 miles. When there is pain, you did too much too soon. The body was not prepared to work as hard, and the muscles were strained to the point of injury.

Exercise can be a wellspring of health and restoration or a source of severe harm, depending on its application.

Let me explain the risk of arthritis.

Imagine that the muscles repeatedly work far harder than they're capable of. The muscles aren't strong enough to hold up the weights at this time. Along with tearing up more muscle tissue than necessary, heavy weights pull on the joints. The joints become overloaded. Joints are delicate structures that can be worn down, damaged or torn. Excessive muscular soreness leads to excessive tightness. Excessive tightness creates a very strong pull on the joints, since muscles attach from one bone to another by crossing a joint. Imagine the joint was strained by heavy weights, and now tight muscles pull on it for days to come. The joints will crack loudly in protest when you try to move. Over time, such joint abuse is likely to create arthritis. Arthritis sets in years later. You won't remember which boot camp caused it.

Boot camps can be a great tool for weight loss as long as you have a solid foundation of muscle mass and you don't get sore. Beginners should not attend boot camps. Yes, this is a conservative approach to fitness, and you may hate it and toss this book aside. Getting in the best shape of your life in three months is an unbeatable selling point, but an unethical approach for a company or boot camp to make, in my opinion.

Bragging about or striving for major soreness is more common for men. The warrior comes home, proudly showing off his battle wounds after defeating the enemy. Yet, I have seen my share of competitive professional women who approach the gym and their bodies like a battlefield, seeking glorious victory over their physical limitations. When I refused to push them into maximum soreness boot camp-style, they perceived their sessions as a waste of time and quit.

Don't dance to this 1980s tune.

Taking pride in getting sore at the gym is like bragging about buying a two-seater plane and climbing in without instruction. You get it off the ground, cruise around, and then you crash it because you had no clue how to fly. If you live to tell your story, you say, "Boy, did I ever fly this plane! There's nothing left of it!"

All the while, the rest of us are thinking, "Well, maybe you should have gotten a pilot's license before you got in? Taken a few classes, or read the owner's manual, at least?"

You get the point. We'll cover gauging intensity in the chapter on weight training. You'll learn how to identify your ideal starting weights, and how to increase the load safely so you'll experience consistent change without risking injury.

Have you met your muscles in person yet, and do you know them by name? When gauging intensity, you'll need to be intimately familiar with each muscle group so you can pay attention for feedback from your body. If you know your muscles and their location, your body awareness increases. Paying attention to the sensations in the various muscle groups will aid in restoring your relationship with your body.

LET'S LEARN LATIN:
THE MAJOR MUSCLE GROUPS

This is a bit dry, but you need to know your muscle groups. I don't want to throw Latin words at you if you've no clue where the foreign thing is located. We'll stick with the general area when discussing exercises, but you need to know which ones are triceps or biceps, quadriceps and hamstrings, so you're clear on what muscle you're targeting and paying close attention to.

There are nine major muscle groups. For the sake of simplicity, we will treat the "core" as one muscle group. It'll make it easier to remember the blue print of a full body workout, which you'll find in the Basic Workout.

Technically, the core consists of three separate muscle groups. These are the agonist, antagonist and supporting muscles of your midsection—or the abdominals, the lower back muscles and the obliques around your waist. The core is your center of gravity, the origin and balancing point of all movement, and the supporting structure on which the entire weight of the upper body rests.

Core: **Abdominals:** Rectus abdominus (the stomach muscles)

Back Extensors: Erector spinae (small muscles around your lumbar spine above the pelvis)

Obliques: Abdominal muscles at your waist

Chest: Pectoralis major

Back: Latissimus dorsi

Triceps: Triceps brachii (back or outer portion of the upper arm)

Biceps: Biceps brachii (top or inner portion of the upper arm)

Shoulder: Deltoid

Quadriceps: Quadriceps femoris (top of the thigh)

Hamstrings: Biceps femoris (back of the thigh)

Calf: Soleus or Gastrocnemius

RESPECT THE LAWS OF ARCHITECTURE: WORK ALL NINE MAJOR MUSCLE GROUPS

If your body is your temple and the home of your eternal spirit, you want that temple to be built by a skilled architect. Amateurs need not apply. You want your temple to be built so solidly that it can withstand an earthquake, and the roof shouldn't collapse during stormy weather. When exercising, you need to think like an architect or the structure will eventually cave in.

Your musculoskeletal frame is your temple's foundation. The bones, muscles, ligaments and joints of upper and lower body are interconnected and stabilized by the core. The more solid your foundation, the better and longer it will hold up. A solid foundation requires that all structural elements support each other at an ideal ratio.

The heart needs to be strong enough to circulate oxygen and the oxygen intake through the lungs needs to be optimal, which can be accomplished by cardiovascular training.

When lifting weights, you must build up and maintain all nine major muscle groups to create a lasting structure. If you are to play favorites, pick the core. As the center of gravity, core strength provides the most stability to your structure.

Exercising all nine major muscle groups is the most essential and yet the most unknown factor in weight training. At any gym, on any given day, you can observe the majority of gym patrons working away heartily at providing orthopedic surgeons and physical therapists with future patients. If you listen closely, you may even hear the chorus of bragging about sports injuries.

Performing random mismatched exercises does more harm than good.

Since all structural elements of your musculoskeletal foundation are interconnected, exercising select muscle groups while ignoring others will cause muscular imbalances.

For example, working a muscle makes it stronger. When a muscle is stronger, it creates a stronger pull. Now, imagine you worked very hard on your back muscles. Imagine how the stronger back muscles create a stronger pull. What happens? You end up arching backward. If you arch backward, your spine will no longer be straight because its natural alignment derails. A misaligned spine squeezes discs or compresses vertebrae, which results in pain.

A straight spine is a healthy spine. Since muscles work in pairs of agonist and antagonist, you need to work each pair equally. An easier way of imagining agonist and antagonist is envisioning the front and back of your body. The spine is in between the front and back. Work both sides, and the spine will stay in alignment.

The same applies to any joint. Muscles attach from one bone across a joint to another.

Imagine the arm. You can bend it, and you can straighten it. The muscle pair on the upper arm is biceps and triceps. The biceps bends the arm, the triceps straightens it. If one pulls stronger than the other, it will damage the delicate structure of the joint in between the upper and lower arm because upper arm muscles attach to the bones of the lower arm.

Sports injuries result either from overuse, traumatic injury, or most often, muscular imbalance. Muscular imbalance is when one muscle of a pair is stronger than its counterpart.

I call the simple routine I'm going to show you in the practical instruction section the *Basic Workout*, because it gives you one exercise for each of the nine major muscle groups. Think of it as a blueprint for a professional workout. It's a place to start, build from, do variations of, and add exercises to. Every workout routine, no matter how advanced, is only a variation of the Basic Workout.

Remember the major muscle groups, and create your exercise regimens according to the laws of architecture.

BREAKING NEWS:
YOU CAN'T SPOT-REDUCE

A popular myth about weight training will tell you that exercise will shrink an area of your body where you hold weight; your abdomen, for example. Lots of crunches are supposed to melt the fat. Unfortunately, fat won't disappear in the places you build muscle unless you lose weight.

Where you lose fat deposits is genetically determined and there's nothing you can do other than liposuction. Liposuction hurts, is expensive, and the fat deposits often return because your genetic program decides the location is a good choice.

You might ask, why get into bodysculpting if you can't spot reduce? We can't sculpt fat, but we can sculpt muscle. We can make muscle bigger, smaller or add the personal touch of a shape we desire.

Fat may sit stubbornly on top of beautifully sculpted muscle, but you can't see the muscular cuts until the fat deposit decreases.

Luckily, muscle fiber is smaller and denser than fat deposits, and building muscle will make your physique tighter. You can be a plus-sized bombshell and tighten your curves into luscious shapes. The fat won't disappear in the areas you worked, but the form will change. Full-figured women with great muscular tone are bigger in size, and a bigger size can look stunning when it's tightened into a Rubenesque work of art.

If you don't like Rubenesque, or you desire a smaller size and want to lose weight, you'll have to work on changing body composition with weight lifting, cardiovascular training, stretching, and dietary change.

EXERCISE IS THE ULTIMATE ANTI-AGING PROGRAM

Once you reach age 30, the body begins its steady decline of physical breakdown. The metabolism slows down due to the gradual loss of muscle mass, and the musculoskeletal frame becomes weaker and more fragile with every decade.

This was acceptable when the average life expectancy was around 40—say, in the early 1900s in the United States—but it's no longer acceptable since we've begun outliving the timelines of our skeletons. The body wasn't meant to last as long as our lives do now!

Nicholas A. DiNubile, an orthopedic surgeon and author of *Frame Work*, writes that you lose four percent of your muscle mass each decade after age 25. After age 40, you lose one percent per year. There are different estimates of how much muscle mass you lose, but I consider his writing and research reliable. Either way, the body's breakdown begins earlier than expected and the consequence is the toll old age takes on our bodies.

Almost everyone understands the practicality of having a retirement fund. Investing in mobility during retirement is less common. Do you still want to be walking when you use that retirement fund? Fragile old age can be avoided with weight training and upkeep of muscle mass. Fragility is the result of weakness. Stiffness is the result of lost flexibility. Fragile old age is not natural, but a consequence of lifestyle choices.

While you can still build muscle past age 90, starting early gives you a protective edge.

Maintaining muscle mass and flexibility will save you from back, neck, knee and shoulder problems, which can become severe enough that surgery is the last resort. Many back and knee surgeries can be avoided by maintaining the necessary muscle, since muscle buffers movement and protects the spine and joints. Most back issues can be remedied effectively with correct exercise. Most knee problems can be improved significantly, as well.

A Swedish study explored the difference between chronological and biological age in relation to fertility. Chronological age is the number of years that have passed since your birth. Biological age is the estimated age of your muscles, bones, organs, and brain. The study found increased fertility in very fit women between the ages of 40 and 50. Biologically, these women's organs were younger than the unconditioned and out of shape control group. You won't simply feel better or even younger, but your body will age less rapidly.

There are current studies about possibly better cognitive skills in seniors who exercise compared to those who don't, due to the increased blood flow to the brain. These studies are still inconclusive, but it's worth considering. Improved blood flow to the brain means more oxygen. Oxygen is the energy miracle drug. Stay tuned for the studies when they conclude.

Starting early and continuing to build lean muscle mass will also make you leaner with advancing decades. Imagine getting leaner and more sensuous as you age! Imagine enjoying your physicality in your sixties, versus expecting to be finished with life as a woman because your good years are supposedly over.

For some of us, our values will shift as we age and we may find more fulfillment nurturing the next generation, rather than seeking enjoyment in living in a beautiful body. But what if the old paradigms are shifting and we can continue enjoying our physicality far past the time previous generations did?

"Old and tired" is so last century. We have new role models who redefine what aging can look like.

Jack LeLanne, the godfather of bodybuilding, worked out for an hour and a half every day at age ninety-five. After that, he went for a half-hour swim. At 61, he entertained himself one fine afternoon by pulling 10 boats with 77 passengers for more than a mile. He swam in handcuffs and it took less than an hour. (Why handcuffs? Makes me wonder where his mind was.)

In a 2015 *Harper's Bazaar* edition, Sharon Stone's body at 58 made 20-year-olds weep with envy. Madonna is leaner in her fifties than she was in her twenties, because she spent her time adding muscle instead of losing it. Jack, Sharon, and Madonna made investments that reaped high returns. They are not the only ones. There are many other examples, not all of them A-listers.

The breakdown we associate with growing old begins at age 30. Don't put up with it. You can be old at age 35, or you can be in top shape in your eighties. Once, a woman in her mid-eighties told me she was going on a skiing trip—down-slope, not cross country. How you age is partially genetic, but a lot of it is choice. Nicholas A. DiNubile stated that a 60-year-old can outperform a 20-year-old, given the 60-year-old is well-conditioned and the

20-year-old is not.

Everyone who defies age by training their minds and bodies updates the collective belief system about how limited we should be at any given age. Be a role model for those who come after you by keeping up your strength.

REALISTIC GOALS EQUALS LESS FRUSTRATION

Being in the best shape of your life within three months is a realistic goal for those who have spent at least one diligent year at the gym, building a solid foundation of muscle mass. For everyone else, it's unrealistic and potentially harmful. Unrealistic expectations will leave you even more frustrated with your body.

When setting goals, remember that the body is your temple. Do you want to build a temple or a McMansion? A McMansion may be faster to build, but a temple lasts longer. If you were going to hire an architect for the job, you'd have to be specific about what kind of structure you want.

We don't build McMansions in this book. We build temples. When you get ready to build, you need to think like an architect.

Architects build in phases, one phase after another. In exercise science, these phases are called cycles. The first cycle for beginners or anyone returning to exercise after an extended leave of absence is building a strong foundation of full body muscle mass. Another component of building the foundation can be changing body composition.

Changing body composition is the action of decreasing body fat while increasing muscle mass. The two processes complement each other beautifully and happen naturally when you combine weight lifting and cardiovascular exercise. Against common belief, you don't need to lose weight before you build muscle. I hope you've stuck with me long enough to understand that increasing metabolism is a priority.

Building the foundation means exercising all nine major muscle groups equally. You'll prevent injury and pain by avoiding muscular imbalance, and you'll slow down the aging process.

A solid foundation is flexible. There could be an earthquake. The building needs to be able to bend for sudden shocks and shakes, which will surely happen eventually. Flexibility training must be part of any building and maintenance cycle.

After building a solid foundation, you can move on to beautifying your building. Think of it this way: It makes little sense to apply pretty stucco to the ceiling before the roof is finished.

How long should you work on your first cycle?

It depends on your personal goals and the time you're willing to dedicate. Three months minimum is a safe bet. Six months is average, and nine to twelve months is a good choice if you're starting past the age of 45 and want to minimize wear and tear on your musculoskeletal frame.

Let me explain what I mean by building McMansions. These are the exercise regimens that promise you'll be in the best shape of your life within three months. It's a great selling point for underemployed personal trainers, boot camps, magazines and the like, but the damage to the musculoskeletal frame is not worth the instant gratification. If you participate in such programs, you'll see changes but they will be temporary and flimsy. You won't have a solid structure because you'll have no foundation. A beginner will never have the same muscular definition after six to nine weeks of boot camp than someone who has spent a year building lean mass. A beginner attempting to exercise at the same intensity as an advanced fitness buff will likely be working on future arthritis. Don't spend your time hurting yourself, no matter your reasoning.

Spend three to six months on building your foundation. You will feel better and more present in your body after your first workout, and your sense of well-being will increase with every session. There's no need to rush. Enjoy your body and experience the sensation of awakening muscle and increased circulation. Take pleasure in heightened physical awareness and your growing sensual expression. Don't rush just so you can look good for someone else at the expense of your temple.

In your advanced cycles, you can begin to sculpt. It's the beautifying process. You'll have enough lean muscle mass as material which you can sculpt, and you'll know how to emphasize muscle groups without doing harm.

Eventually, you'll like your architectural work of art, and you will enter the maintenance phase.

Time commitments need to be realistic and sustainable. If they are not, you'll put off getting started because you don't have time or you'll quit because it takes too much time.

For best results, work the entire body with weights three times per week. Rest 48 hours between weight lifting sessions. Weight lifting on Monday, Wednesday, and Friday is a standard example. If you can't bear the idea of going to the gym three times per week, try two times per week. You'll progress more slowly and changes will be less dramatic, but you'll still see a difference.

Always start with a five to 10 minute warm-up, and end with five to 10 minutes of stretching.

Work all nine major muscle groups three times per week. Perform three to four sets for each major muscle group.

TIME COMMITMENT

In the beginning, when you need to move slowly to prevent dizziness and feeling out of breath, a weight lifting session should take approximately 45 minutes. A general guideline for weight lifting sessions is 30 to 60 minutes, depending on your personal preference. Warming up and stretching time are extra, which adds 10 to 20 minutes.

If you are in the beginning cycle and want to split routines, you can also shorten the time commitment per session. Let's say you want to split the workout into upper body one day, then lower body the next day. If you're building your foundation and you want to work all nine major muscle groups three times per week, you'll need to get to the gym six days per week.

Lifting weights six times per week is great for increasing metabolism and reducing the daily time commitment to 30 minutes. However, once the initial enthusiasm wears off, six days at the gym can be dreadful. If you started at six days per week and you can't sustain it, switch to two to three times per week. Over-commitment frequently leads to under-achievement. I haven't seen many clients who kept up the pace of going to the gym almost every day.

Once you're in an advanced stage and in great cardiovascular condition, you can use circuit-training, which means you hop seamlessly from one exercise to another to work all nine major muscle groups. Instead of resting between sets, you switch muscle groups and work one muscle while another rests. For example, you shift back and forth between chest and back exercises until you have completed three to four sets for each. When you know your exercise routine very well, you can circulate the gym and do one set for each muscle group until you've worked the entire body. This can cut the time commitment of weight lifting to 30 minutes per session.

If the time commitment still seems dreadful, remember that fitness runs its course in cycles. First you build the foundation, then you keep building and sculpting, and finally you enter the maintenance phase.

Maintenance is when you love your work of art and the building phase is over. Maintenance takes less work than building. You can switch to working all nine major muscle groups two times per week and get the job done in 30 to 45 minutes, but you'll need to lift heavier. You'll already be used to it, so it won't be too difficult to increase weights. The heavier you lift, the longer muscles need for recovery. You'll utilize the longer recovery phases to reduce time commitment.

Circuit-training is the most high-performing choice for the maintenance phase of your ideal physique and for keeping your weight where you want it to be. Circuit-training is a low time commitment while it burns calories at a very high rate and sky-rockets your metabolism. Lift heavy and move fast.

But please, don't do it as a beginner, unless you don't mind mouth-to-mouth CPR on the gym floor because you passed out. High-intensity exercise for the unconditioned beginner can lead to heart attacks.

Let's talk time commitment for cardiovascular training.

Cardiovascular training can be done almost daily. You're not causing microscopic injury to the muscles, and the muscles don't need recovery time to grow. If you want to kick start your metabolism and lose weight, consider six times at 20 to 30 minutes per week. Short, daily sessions are most effective for your metabolism and changing metabolic baseline.

Two hours on the treadmill once a week is very ineffective for both heart and metabolism. A long exercise session once a week is likely to do more harm than good, because you overload unconditioned joints.

Cardiovascular training utilizes hip and knee joints. Too much of a good thing can become less of a good thing. Give yourself at least one day off from exercise even if you are an exercise maniac. Don't overuse your joints.

Using cardiovascular equipment is better than running in nature. This may be hard to hear for anyone who loves to exercise outside, but I'm speaking from almost two decades of experience with personal training and a prior decade of professional dance training. I haven't come across anyone past their fifties who could still regularly run on hard ground without experiencing knee problems. Cardio equipment provides less impact on joints than hard ground does. There are only a few genetically lucky individuals who can handle running in nature for a lifetime without developing joint problems.

If you're looking for a time effective exercise routine, I suggest three weight lifting sessions per week combined with 10 minutes of cardiovascular training before weight lifting, and an additional

10 minutes afterward. This way, you utilize the warm-up phase as your first half of cardiovascular training. Breaking up the routines can make the experience less dreadful.

If the time commitment still seems like more than you can possibly bear, I have another great idea.

Go to the gym for two to three weight lifting sessions per week, and keep them short. Throw in abdominal exercises at work or at home whenever you can take a break. Buy a piece of cardiovascular equipment for home use and set it up with a built-in reward, such as watching TV while you work out.

Used cardiovascular equipment is easy to find and ridiculously inexpensive, because the owner meant to use it, didn't use it, and can't wait to get rid of the evidence of their shame. Stationary bicycles or elliptical walkers for home use are often very small and light, so you can fit it into a small apartment or put it in a closet when you're done. I have yet to come across a client who hasn't lost weight after she bought a piece of home cardio equipment and set it up with a reward. My stationary bicycle is set up so I have an excuse to watch German movies. "Hey, I can't do the dishes right now. I have to finish my exercise session."

PART 2: THEORETICAL INSTRUCTION

CHAPTER 1

CARDIOVASCULAR TRAINING – NEED MORE ENERGY, ANYONE?

What is the purpose of cardiovascular training? Let's do a quick repeat, so you have all the facts in one place. You'll be familiar with the basic ideas from previous chapters. I don't mean to bore you, but I want you to be an expert architect when building your structure so you'll have the edge of a professional. You'll build solid beauty for a lifetime, not for a short-lived event.

Cardiovascular training trains the heart and cardiovascular system.

If you run up the stairs and your heart rate skyrockets, leaving you gasping for air, your heart is weak. A weak heart has to contract quickly and many times to move blood and oxygen from the lungs into the tissue, where oxygen is needed when you exert yourself. You're gasping for air to get enough oxygen into the lungs and into the blood stream, which typically doesn't work very well and feels unpleasant. You may even get lightheaded, and if you are older, you may need a moment of rest until the heart manages to distribute oxygen.

If frequent exercise requires the heart to work harder, it becomes stronger. It's a muscle, after all. A stronger heart contracts more forcefully and doesn't need to contract as often to get the work done. You run up the stairs and the powerful heart muscle shoots oxygen where it belongs.

During the 1970s, popular belief suggested that anyone past age 40 shouldn't exert themselves as much to protect their heart. Today, we think the opposite. Make sure to exert the heart regularly so it keeps working. Exert the heart at low to medium intensity, the kind you can keep up for long periods of time.

Since the body responds to demand in order to secure survival, it will build more capillaries (tiny blood vessels) so the blood can deliver oxygen to tissue in need. More oxygen circulating throughout the body feels like a surge of energy. If you maintain cardiovascular fitness, you'll have more energy every day. A person in their sixties can have significantly more energy than a person in their forties.

If you exercise regularly, the body grows more capillaries (tiny blood vessels) so that the blood can deliver oxygen more quickly into the tissue where it's needed. The heart becomes stronger and can keep up the job more effectively. A stronger heart moves blood and oxygen with less beats per minute, because the beats are more powerful. The heart no longer races when you run up the stairs, because it distributes oxygen in a few smooth moves. Increased oxygen consumption is the pro-word for the physical change that results in the feeling of fitness. Oxygen is the miracle substance that fuels us with energy. A weak heart and lower oxygen consumption is what makes us feel like an old, wet, moldy towel.

Cardiovascular training is best combined with stretching. Your hamstrings, hip flexors, and lower back will become tight from running or cycling. Let's discuss how it's done.

HOW'S IT DONE?

The heart is a delicate thing and since it's a muscle, it needs to be trained like one. Muscles like gradual progressive overload. They like a challenge to work a little harder than usual, and they like rest afterward so they can grow. They prefer consistency. Growth is a process, not an event. To train the heart or any other muscle, you need to start easy, be steady, and increase the workload gently over time.

Here is how to start a cardiovascular exercise routine:

First week: 3 days, 15 to 20 minutes per day. Take it easy. Slow down if it's uncomfortable.

Second week: 3 days, 15 to 20 minutes per day. Speed it up a little. Stay comfortable.

Third week: 3 to 5 days, 15 to 30 minutes per day. Speed it up a bit more. Make it more challenging by increasing the resistance on the equipment so you pedal harder.

Fourth week: 3 to 6 days, 15 to 30 minutes per day. Keep building. A bit longer, faster, and more challenging.

The above is only an outline to give you a general idea. However, you get better results by exercising less time but more frequently versus exercising an hour once or twice a week. 20 minutes a day is better than an hour once a week.

Why? Because the heart is a muscle. Muscles like consistency. They like a bit of challenge, rest, and over time, increased challenge. Consistency is key.

Cardio will only feel hard and uncomfortable if you are doing too much too soon. It'll feel like running up or down the stairs to chase your dog, your child, or your significant other. Your heart beats like crazy, you gasp for air, and you get nauseous or lightheaded. Your legs feel like lead, and five minutes turn into eternity.

In contrast, if you exercise regularly at a comfortable pace, you will become stronger without noticing. The training will continue to feel easy, even though you keep speeding it up. It will feel like the release of pent-up energy—*not* like an unpleasant strain.

HOW TO ADVANCE

Once you've reached a comfortable level of cardiovascular fitness as part of your routine, here's a general guideline for continuing to build cardiovascular fitness:

Start cardiovascular training with a warm-up phase. Exercise at a comfortable pace for the first five to 10 minutes.

After that, increase the speed in *five minute* increments. If your total training time is 20 minutes, increase your cardiovascular fitness by picking up speed after five to 10 minutes, increase the speed in five minute increments, and slow down after 15 minutes.

If you want to keep your training time at 20 minutes total but increase the challenge to the cardiovascular system, you can increase the resistance of the equipment. This will increase the heart rate and load on the leg muscles.

If you want to train for more than twenty minutes, increase total training time by five minutes per week. While this may be a slow approach to advancement, it minimizes stress on the joints. Don't go from 10 minutes of training to 45 minutes or an hour.

Once you are advanced and well-conditioned, you can safely increase total training time by 10 minute increments.

The final five minutes are the *cool-off* period. Return to the comfortable pace, and slow it down every minute.

HOW TO BURN FAT

Cardiovascular training burns stored sugars first, and then turns to fat storages. It's a survival issue. You may be hunting and stalking your prey for long periods of time, or you may be migrating to make sure your herds find enough foliage to snack on. Either way, you need an energy source that will keep you going for a long time. Fat storages provide energy during low intensity activity for long periods of time.

It's unlikely that you're chasing prey on a treadmill. However, the body doesn't know this. You might as well trick it into believing you are, and get it to utilize fat storages.

If you want to be scientific about it, here is an ideal training zone to access fat storages. The formula is:

Cardiovascular Training – Need More Energy, Anyone?

220 minus the age of the person.

Then train at 55 percent to 65 percent of that amount.

220 minus your age gives you the maximum amount of beats per minute your heart can handle.

Around 60 percent of that amount is the ideal fat burning zone. Monitor your heart rate during cardiovascular exercise. Most equipment has this function on the handlebars. If not, take your pulse. Don't fall off the treadmill if you do.

If you don't want to do the math, and you don't want to take your pulse, make it easy on yourself. Exercise at a speed at which you could still talk if you had to, but you'd rather not. The breath should become deeper and more even. If you no longer feel like chatting with your treadmill neighbor, but you're not going so fast that it's a short sprint, you're most likely in the ideal fat burning zone.

Another sign of the fat burning zone is sweating. If you don't sweat after 20 minutes, you're either a beginner and still adjusting to exercise, or you're too slow.

The ability to sweat is an adaptation to exercise. It shows that the body has "learned" to cool itself off through sweating. However, after a month of regular cardiovascular training, you should be able to sweat. If you are not sweating, you are too slow.

Should you always aim for the fat burning zone?

It depends on your goals. If you want to reduce body fat, yes. If you're exercising for general health, you can also stay within this zone. If your goal is increasing metabolism, no. Increasing metabolism requires you go as fast as you can or throw in short sprints.

Burning fat happens at low to medium intensity. Increasing metabolism happens at high intensity.

Both work for losing weight. Training in the fat burning zone leads to weight loss if you train consistently and reduce your calorie intake. Increasing metabolism is the longer road to weight loss because the body's metabolic baseline takes time to adjust, but an increased metabolism makes it easier to keep the weight off.

Burning fat is not the same as burning calories.

Burning fat means you're using up your long-term energy storages, also called fat deposits. To do so, you need to use up the currently circulating energy in your system first. Currently circulating energy consists of the calories you took in during the day. If weight loss is your goal, you need to lower daily calorie intake, so there is a need to use up long-term energy storages in fat deposits. Fat burning happens after you use up your daily calories.

Burning calories means you're using up the currently circulating energy, also called your daily calorie intake. The calories are stored sugars which are readily available for immediate energy.

If you want to burn off a particularly mean Thanksgiving dinner or giant piece of cake, exercise at a high speed to burn off calories so they're not stored as fat.

Low- to medium-intensity cardio draws from fat storages after using up stored sugars.

High-intensity cardio burns up stored sugars (calories) and increases metabolism.

HOW OFTEN DO YOU NEED TO TRAIN?

For weight loss, do 20 to 30 minutes of cardiovascular training six times per week or as often as you can. For general health and fitness, do 20 to 30 minutes three times per week. For increasing metabolism, long-term weight loss or weight maintenance, do 20 to 30 minutes six times per week or as often as you can.

Twenty minutes every day will do more for shifting your metabolism into higher gear and for improving the health of your heart than an occasional hour. The body burns more calories after exercise. Energy consumption peaks right after exercise, and then decreases slowly. Even 12 hours after exercise, the energy consumption is still higher; you still burn more calories than before your exercise session.

Daily cardiovascular exercise "jump starts" your metabolism until the body becomes used to it and adopts it as a new baseline.

Remember to take one day off every week.

It'll be your designated day of productive rest. Lounge around proudly. Your body needs recovery time. Remind yourself that exercising every day is for amateurs and true athletes honor rest.

Increasing the metabolism through the use of cardiovascular

exercise does require some patience. For women, it takes eight to 12 weeks of regular exercise to make a noticeable difference. For men, it's a little faster.

TIMING: WHEN IS THE BEST TIME TO TRAIN?

Cardiovascular exercise in the morning is the most popular and intuitive choice. It makes sense to begin your day actively and keep it going. However, cardiovascular exercise in the evening after dinner is most effective for weight loss.

Exercising in the morning increases metabolism for the rest of the day, which is a good but not a great choice. Theoretically, you will lose weight as long as you consume (use up) more energy than you took in. But morning exercise may make you hungrier as calories are used up faster, and you may eat more throughout the day. Monitoring clients for almost two decades has shown me that evening exercise is far more effective.

You can maintain your ideal weight or exercise for general health by exercising in the morning, but avoid doing so for weight loss.

Evening or after dinner exercise burns the calories of the day. After exercise, the metabolic rate is elevated, meaning you'll burn more calories during the night. Since you won't be eating during the night, there's a higher chance you'll burn more than you took in. Using the afterburn during sleep is effective for weight loss. So is using up the consumed calories of the day.

You may need to trudge to the gym after dinner, or have dinner after work and before you go to the gym. If you own cardio equipment for home use, you can create an afterburn before you go to sleep.

Some clients report difficulty falling asleep after exercise. Usually, it's temporary and the body will adjust to evening exercise within two weeks. If not, pay close attention to how long you need to relax after exercise, and find your own comfort zone.

Try late afternoon or lunch hour exercise. Lunch hour exercise is great if you consumed the majority of calories for breakfast and lunch, and your afternoon snack or dinner will be small.

If you are a stay-at-home mom battling post-pregnancy weight, you can do both morning and evening exercise, or increase your metabolism with three to four bouts of 10 to 15 minute cardio sessions on home equipment.

As a general guideline, exercise after you consumed the majority of your daily calories and losing weight will become easier. In general, avoid exercise first thing in the morning. Give your body an hour minimum to wake up through gentle movement. Joints are not yet lubricated. Muscles are cold, collagen is stiff. Discs between spinal vertebrae are not yet compressed by the forces of gravity. Your risk of injury is highest in the morning or after long periods of inactivity.

CHAPTER 2

WEIGHT TRAINING: WEIGHTS ARE THE FRIEND WHO WON'T LET YOU DOWN

Let's review the most important facts. Alternatively, you can skip this section if you're certain you don't need it.

Weight training builds muscle, also referred to as lean mass. Building or maintaining muscle increases strength and muscular endurance, and it increases your metabolism. Simply put, increased muscle mass burns more calories than less muscle. If you have more lean mass, the body consistently burns more calories because it needs the extra energy to sustain its basic functions.

After the age of 30, the body begins a steady decline of breaking down lean mass. With every decade, you get weaker. What's worse, with every decade you also need less calories, because the body needs less energy to sustain itself. Less lean mass requires fewer calories. The result is a steady increase of body fat.

You have several choices. Either you live on a strict low-carbohydrate diet, or you exercise like mad. Neither one is a good choice, because extreme lifestyle changes rarely last. The best you can do is defy the aging process by building and maintaining lean muscle mass, and adjusting your dietary intake in moderation. A balanced combination of both will give you a higher than average metabolism as compared with your age group and you'll also maintain your strength.

Lifting heavier weights can burn up to 700 calories an hour. Also, the afterburn (increased energy consumption) after weight training is substantially high.

The goal is increasing the metabolism and establishing a new comfort zone. Bodies form habits. If the body becomes accustomed to jump-starting its metabolism, it will adopt a new base rate. Building and maintaining lean mass gives the body a major tune-up.

Remember the dare of lifting heavy? Go ahead and try it. Lift "heavy." Build up slowly and safely, and see if you like what happens. If not, you can always lighten up. Gaining muscle is much harder than losing it.

HOW TO BUILD A MUSCLE

Building a muscle safely requires understanding the concept of Gradual Progressive Overload.

Overload means you're working every muscle group slightly harder than it's used to. Progressive means you'll continue to work the muscle harder and harder over time. Gradual means you'll take care to do it slowly enough that the muscle can adapt to the stress by growing.

If you build muscle progressively, the muscles will lift only slightly more than they can handle and they will adjust without pulling too heavily on the joints.

Additionally, when you lift progressively higher weights, the body responds by storing more calcium in the bones. Weight-bearing exercises are very effective for the prevention and treatment of Osteoporosis.

Challenge the muscle just slightly past its comfort zone. When you do, you create a microscopic injury. If you let it rest for 48 hours, the muscle will heal. After it's healed, do it again.

Because we're designed for survival, the muscle will respond to ongoing demand by growing. After all, it wants to be prepared for next time. Your survival may depend on being able to meet the increased physical challenge.

The key is consistency. If you challenge the muscle once a month, it'll still heal, but it won't grow. Growth only happens as an adaption to ongoing demand. You need to trick the body into perceiving muscular growth as essential to your survival.

If you go to the gym in a moment of madness and tear your muscles down by lifting too heavily, you'll crawl home and limp the next day. If you can still walk, that is. You will have an injury. You will need time to heal, longer than 48 hours. The muscle will heal, but that'll be it. You'll hate how it feels, because it hurts. You can't return to the gym because you're injured, and the body sees no reason to grow muscle because there is no ongoing demand. Injury is responded to by healing. Demand is responded to by growing.

We'll get into gauging intensity in the next chapter. Gauging intensity means figuring out how much to challenge the muscle so you create a microscopic injury, not a major one. It means figuring out your starting weights, and how to keep building.

When building muscle, work in sets.

For a beginner's workout, you'll do three to four sets of 10 to 12 repetitions.

Repetitions are the number of times you repeat a movement. Let's say you start with repeating the movement of the exercise 12 times. That's 12 repetitions.

Your 12 repetitions make up a set. After performing a set, you rest for 30 to 60 seconds. Then you start another round of 12 repetitions, which makes up your second set.

Three sets is the minimum needed to build muscle.

For each muscle group, you need to do at least three sets. You can do more sets, but not less.

Here's another concept you need to know about increasing lean mass. It doesn't apply as much in the beginning cycle, but it's good to be aware of it in the future. It's the concept of Shock-Adaption-Staleness.

You put a shock on the muscle, it adapts to the challenge, and then becomes stale or stagnant. The muscle adapted to the challenge and settled. If survival is secured with a minor adaption, why continue growing? Growing is work. Human beings and bodies are lazy in nature. We only do what we need to do to survive. Otherwise, we can't be bothered, unless there is pleasure involved.

Muscles are similar. The mean little things will only continue growing if they absolutely have to. When working with machines, the muscle is challenged from one specific angle, or with one specific kind of stimulation. If you stick with the exercises you enjoy, you'll limit the results you get. The muscle will only adapt to the stimulation you provide.

The solution is variety. Increase the weights and sets slowly and gradually until you have the lean look you want. Use different machines with different grips and angles, and use free weights to keep challenging the muscles into continuous adaptation. We'll go into more detail in the chapter on Advanced Exercise.

Respect the laws of architecture. The key concept in exercise science is Symmetry. Don't build your house on an uneven foundation. It'll collapse on you eventually.

Muscles work in pairs of Agonist and Antagonist, as discussed earlier. The bicep bends the arm, and the triceps pull it straight. If you work the biceps more than the triceps, the biceps will pull more forcefully on the elbow joint. The joint will wear out and become damaged or misaligned.

If you work the chest more than the back, the chest muscles will pull from the front, creating a hunched over appearance and a humpback. If you work the back more than the chest, the back muscles pull more forcefully and the chest starts to point to the sky. Remember, only a straight spine is a pain-free spine.

Be nice to your joints if you want them to last, and keep your spine straight unless you want frequent dates with your orthopedic surgeon.

HOW HEAVY SHOULD THE WEIGHTS BE?

Gauging intensity makes or breaks your exercise routine. Too much weight creates injury, while too little weight leaves you frustrated and prone to quitting because you see no results.

If you want to build muscle, you need to exhaust the muscle in a short period of time, say 10 to 12 repetitions.

Exhausting the muscle means that the last few repetitions are a bit of a strain, and the very last repetition is the point at which the muscle is about to fail. Muscular failure is when you can't do another repetition without losing correct form.

As you perform the last few repetitions and move toward muscular failure, there should be a burning sensation that increases until the muscle "fails." The burning sensation is frequently perceived as a mild but uncomfortable "pain."

What do you do when lifting weights feels painful? You'll try to avoid it, of course. It's only natural. Not only does it feel unpleasant, but avoiding pain is also a survival instinct. If you cause yourself pain, you might get injured and be unable to run away from predators. Isolating one specific muscle and working it to a point of perceived "pain" goes against survival instinct.

However, chances are small that there are predators at the gym. At least, not the kind that wants to eat you for dinner. But the body doesn't know this, and you need to recondition yourself into tolerating the "pain" that's nothing but a minor burning sensation caused by dropping PH levels in the muscle.

The burning sensation is what makes a muscle. Remember, you want to create a microscopic injury. Microscopic, not major. Creating a microscopic injury is a bit uncomfortable in the beginning, until you are used to it. If you continuously remind yourself that the burning sensation is not a pain and is by no means a threat to your survival, you will eventually become desensitized. Once you are desensitized, you will no longer register a burning sensation.

After the muscle failed, it needs rest. In the beginning cycle, the resting period between sets should be 30 to 60 seconds. If you have moved on to the advanced stages of bodysculpting, working on dramatic cuts or shapes, you may need to rest longer.

You can rest on the equipment you're using, or you can do a set for an opposing muscle group in the meantime. Moving back and forth between working different muscles is a simple version of circuit-training.

If you are able to lift set after set for one muscle group and you don't need to rest, the weight is not heavy enough. Remember, you want to approach muscular failure at the end of each set. If the weight is heavy enough and you need to rest, it's feedback that you're on the right track.

You may notice a slight shaking in your muscles when you begin weight lifting sessions. Shaking isn't feedback that the weights are too heavy; it's a necessary adaptation of your neuromuscular system. Nerve impulses need to register the new activity in the brain. After 10 to 14 days, the neurological traffic jam is sorted out and the movement becomes secure and steady.

To be sure you're working at the ideal intensity, rate the weights during exercise. Then rate your muscles 36 hours after the workout. If you worked with a trainer, the trainer would ask you to do the same and adjust the weight accordingly. Learn to do it yourself, and you'll see professional results.

GAUGING INTENSITY: RATING THE WEIGHTS WITH THE SCALE OF PERCEIVED EXERTION

Sensitivity to workload is more psychological than physical. What you think about lifting determines how heavy it feels. One person may insist the weights aren't difficult but fail at four repetitions when the goal was 12. The next person may complain the weights are too heavy but do three sets without rest or fatigue.

When rating your weights, try to be very honest with yourself. Cheating yourself only leads to disappointment. Or you can exercise with a friend and hold each other accountable, so neither of you lift too lightly.

When performing a set, rate the sensation in the muscle toward the end of the set.

SCALE OF PERCEIVED EXERTION

1. I don't feel anything. (Extremely easy.)

2. I barely feel anything. (Very easy.)

3. I feel something, but it's insignificant. (Quite easy.)

4. I feel that I lifted something. (Somewhat easy.)

5. I feel it. (Increasing intensity.)

6. I feel a workload. (Starting to become work.)

7. I feel a slight strain. (Getting heavy toward the end.)

8. I feel increased strain. (Becoming heavier.)

9. I can barely finish the set. (Very heavy.)

10. I can't finish the set. (Too heavy.)

Let's apply this scale.

In the first two to three weeks, train at a **5** on the Scale of Perceived Exertion.

After three weeks, increase the weights to a **6** on the Scale.

After four weeks, train at **7** to **8** on the Scale, but don't go any heavier.

Once you're advanced, you can work heavy cycles which you rate at a nine to facilitate intense muscular growth. You should build up slowly to heavy cycles, so your muscles are able to handle the strain without getting sore.

GAUGING PROGRESS: USE THE

SENSITIVITY SCALE

You can use this process after your very first weight lifting workout, but ideally after every workout. It will help you fine tune the load and give you feedback when to increase the weights.

For your first workout, use fairly light weights. The weights should be so light that you can comfortably complete three sets of 10 to 12 repetitions without muscular failure or excessive shaking. Complete a full body workout, then go home and listen to your body's response over the next 24 to 36 hours.

If you feel nothing, it wasn't heavy enough.

If it hurts, it was too much.

Of course, there is a gray zone between too heavy and too light and hopefully, your first workout was in this gray zone. When you go home, you will most likely feel as if you did something. You'll feel less stiff and maybe a bit fatigued.

After 24 to 36 hours, you'll receive more feedback from your body. The right intensity of weights feels like the muscles "woke up." You can tell you did some work, and you're aware of the major muscle groups, because you can feel where they are.

You may feel a slight tingling sensation or a minor swelling in the muscles. The sensation you're looking for is increased circulation in the muscle, which shows the muscle has been exerted past its previous capacity and is now being repaired. You should feel pleasant and energized, or slightly fatigued but relaxed.

The muscles may feel sensitive to the touch, but there shouldn't be any pain. If movement is restricted and painful, the weight was too heavy. Soreness is off-limits. Never get sore to a point of pain.

Use the Sensitivity Scale to rate the sensitivity in the muscles 24 to 36 hours after every workout, Rate every muscle group and check that all were worked equally. Every time you feel nothing or hardly anything after a workout, it's feedback to increase the weights by small increments.

This process protects you from injury and increases body awareness, because you begin to "listen" to your muscles.

SENSITIVITY SCALE

1. I don't feel anything.

2. I barely feel anything.

3. I feel something, but it's insignificant.

4. I feel that I was physically active.

5. I feel that I lifted something but it wasn't heavy.

6. I feel the workout and its specific exercises. The muscle is tighter and feels a bit tired, but it feels good.

7. I really worked out! The muscle is slightly swollen, tight and could use a stretch.

8. My body feels somewhat heavy and noticeably tired. The muscle is slightly achy.

9. I'm hurting.

10. Ouch! I can barely move.

In the first two to three weeks, train at a **5** on the Scale.

After three weeks, increase the weights to a **6** on the Scale.

After four weeks, train at a **7** on the Scale.

After eight to 12 weeks or when you are advanced, you can begin training at an **8** on the scale.

HOW OFTEN DO YOU LIFT WEIGHTS?

If you continuously challenge a muscle to work a bit harder than it's used to, it responds by growing to accommodate the demand. The growth process takes 48 hours. The correct balance between work and rest is a schedule of weight lifting every other day.

The ideal weight lifting schedule is Monday, Wednesday, and Friday, or Tuesday, Thursday, and Saturday.

Lifting weights every day is counterproductive, especially if you work the same muscle groups over and over again. Weight lifting breaks down muscle fiber and creates a microscopic injury, which should be just enough to trigger growth. But growth is part of the healing process inside the muscle, and healing requires rest. If you don't allow for rest, the muscle continues its breakdown and becomes weaker. You may even damage it.

The correct resting period is 48 hours.

The weight lifting routine should take 45 to 60 minutes. 45 minutes should be plenty of time to work the entire body, leaving you time to stretch at the end.

Set a realistic schedule you can maintain. If you let too much time pass between workouts—for example, if you only train once a week—the muscle will atrophy again after a growth spurt. The body thinks the challenge was only an isolated event, and the gains are minimal. You'll still feel better and less sluggish, but you won't see a major transformation. Training regularly and consistently is the safe and effective way to go.

CORRECT BREATHING

You're almost ready to get started, and you have a good understanding of the components of a professional workout routine. Let's give the concept of breathing a thought. It may seem like a no-brainer, but it isn't.

You may have noticed that it feels right to hold your breath while you're lifting something heavy. Unfortunately, it isn't. During very heavy lifting, incorrect breathing can be lethal. Breathing is similar to delivering gasoline to the engine because muscles need oxygen to perform. Correct breathing takes a good amount of practice to get it right.

Improper breathing can spike blood pressure as high as 480/360. Healthy blood pressure is around 120/80. High spikes in blood pressure can lead to confusion, fainting, and in the worst case, heart attacks.

- Breathe out on the exertion.

- Every time it's heavy, breathe out.

- When you prepare to lift, breathe in first, then breathe out as you are lifting.

If you choose to hold or strain your breath during lifting, you may burst alveoli. Alveoli are the microscopic endings of the bronchial branches, a bit like tiny air sacs. You'll feel a disconcerting chest pain the next day, not harmful but uncomfortable enough to want to avoid it. I've heard of gym patrons who have checked into emergency rooms because they mistook burst alveoli for an impending heart attack. Avoid the scare and don't hurt yourself at the gym.

THE RIGHT GRIP

Always use a closed over- or under-hand grip when lifting weights. For a closed hand grip, four fingers of one hand wrap around the weight or machine handlebar, and the thumb closes around the bottom of the grip.

This may seem self-explanatory, but it isn't, since free weights or handlebars can appear too wide to close the hand comfortably. However, caution is wise and worth the effort. An experienced bodybuilder once told me he dropped dumbbells on his head during a strenuous workout. They had slipped from his sweaty, open-handed grip. He told me of his accident after returning from the hospital.

Using workout gloves is a good idea, since gloves protect the median and carpal tunnel nerves of the hand, and prevent excessive calluses. Gloves secure the grip, so you don't need to grasp the weights too hard. Grasping weights with great tension can overwork the smaller hand muscles and lead to tightness and discomfort. Not grasping weights can lead to dropping them. You get the idea. Close the hand and use gloves.

THE WARM-UP

For both cardiovascular and weight training, the warm-up period is crucial. Never lift weights or stretch without a prior warm-up. Collagen in the muscle is heat dependent, meaning it will only elongate when warm. Pulling on a cold muscle during a stretch is asking for injury. Lifting weights without a warm-up is equally likely to produce injury. Cracking limbs are not a sign of a good stretch but the sound of excessive force on unprepared joints.

The goal of a warm-up is to increase flood flow and metabolic activity in the tissue and lubricate the joints. The minimum for a safe and effective warm-up is five to10 minutes of cardiovascular activity. Start light and move to moderate. In other words, start by walking and speed it slowly until you feel your temperature and heartbeat increasing.

On those tired days, the days when you really don't want to exercise at all, a 20-minute warm-up can work miracles. Once you increase oxygen transport throughout the system, you'll feel energized. It sounds quite unlikely, but it always works.

When you use heavy weights during a more advanced cycle, you may want to add warm-up sets to the cardio warm-up. For warm-up sets, reduce the weights by 50 percent, and perform one to two sets of 15 to 20 repetitions before you move on to heavier sets. This practice is most important during the winter or if you exercise in a heavily air-conditioned environment. Big, muscular men often prefer robustly icy exercise spaces as if they couldn't tolerate a sweat, when heat and sweating actually increase the pliability and performance of muscle tissue.

The heavier you work, the higher the risk of injury. The more warmed up you are, the lower the risk of injury. Injury includes the slow and unnoticed wear and tear of the joints that leads to chronic conditions. Make sure you're warm, not cold. Breaking a sweat is good for you.

If you performed heavy sets during an advanced workout and the joints are stiff the following day, the warm-up was insufficient and needs to be increased.

THE COOL-DOWN

The cool-down period is the last part of the workout and designed to decrease heart rate before you walk out and get into your car. Lifting heavily with steam coming from your nostrils and quitting suddenly can surprise you with a dizzy spell, which is not conducive to keeping your driver's license and your life.

Also, heavy workouts accumulate lactic acid in the muscle

tissue, a byproduct of energy exchange. Muscular soreness can be avoided by performing 10 to 15 minutes of light to moderate cardiovascular activity, during which the lactic acid is recycled for energy. A low intensity cardiovascular cool-down is the smart choice after a strenuous leg workout but can also help after a high intensity full body routine.

The cool-down period is the most sensible time to stretch. Muscle tissue is prepared, collagen is warm and ready to elongate. Stretching gains are greatest in this state and don't compromise joints, tendons, and ligaments. You can cool down for five to 10 or 30 minutes, depending on your goals. If increased flexibility is a goal or dire necessity, stretching every day is most effective. Use the cool-down after weightlifting as your most intense stretching session but add shorter stints of stretching to your daily routine. Warmed up, that is.

CHAPTER 3

STRETCHING: BEAUTY IS GRACEFUL

Cats are elegant. Tree sloths are not. We don't think of elephants as graceful, either. What are you, and what do you want to be?

How you carry yourself is determined by how you move. Graceful movement at any size is appealing to the eye; it is sensual and beautiful. How you move depends greatly on your flexibility.

The beauty of physical expression emerges from interplay of flexibility, good posture and fine-tuned sensory-motor skills.

The way you move and carry your body is read as non-verbal communication, providing clues about your personality.

Hunched shoulders communicate poor self-esteem, even though the cause may be weak chest muscles and a tight upper back. Short steps can communicate impatience, uptightness or childishness, even though the gait is caused by tight hamstrings. Slow moves can be misread as depression, even though the cause may be a tight lower back.

Dancers are perceived as sexually active at any age. Athletes are perceived as strong even if their minds aren't.

Your degree of flexibility and your movement tells volumes

about you which may not be accurate. It may make you appear less life-loving than you really are, or far more insecure. Your movement may have become frozen at a certain time in life when you battled tension and stress, and you may still move the same way as you haven't taken the time to loosen up.

Beauty is graceful. Physical grace happens when you return to your body to strengthen it, recover balance and fine motor skills through exercise, and when you stretch into the fullness of who you are. When you stretch your body into its full range of motion, you are likely to experience the psychological metaphor of expansion. For some reason, it works. You'll feel psychologically larger and less limited if your body is able to move freely.

Let's explore the consequence of inflexibility in detail.

Inflexibility is another word for stiffness. Once you call it stiffness, it's clear why it's an uncomfortable state of being. If you are stiff, there is less range of motion. Two bones connected by a muscle that crosses a joint allow for less movement. Your steps are shorter, your gestures limited. You can only move within your allotted range of motion. You may not have given it much thought, but from the perspective of a dancer, you're caught in a body that doesn't give you a lot of freedom.

With increasing age, you become stiffer. The physical aging process begins at 30 years of age. Collagen becomes brittle and breaks down, while joints produce less lubrication. However, not all loss of flexibility can be blamed on aging.

Think of lifelong Yogis, who can be more flexible in their nineties than the average college student. How you age is partially genetic, but is also affected by lifestyle choices. Without intervention, you'll enter a continuous physical decline at the age of 30. You'll get weaker, less energetic, and stiff.

Stiff muscles are tight. A tight muscle can be pulled and injured more easily through rash movement. With advancing age, the risk of injury increases, just because you are stiff.

Don't despair if you are inflexible and have been as long as you can remember. It's never too late to change the condition of your body, as long as you are willing to be thorough and consistent. Achieving flexibility is easy and requires a low time commitment. As little as 10 minutes a day can restore your flexibility.

Let's look at a few options.

Yoga is a great choice for achieving and maintaining flexibility. It's less ideal for building strength and it certainly won't do much for losing weight. It also won't increase your bone density, because Yoga is low impact on the bones. But it can maintain flexibility into old age. If you're willing to attend Yoga classes two to three times a week, you're making a great investment in your mobility.

For best results, stretch daily. You can alternate between Yoga and gym sessions if your goal is strength and flexibility or if you are willing to exercise daily. If your goal is weight loss, I suggest you postpone Yoga sessions until you're happy with your size and focus on weight loss for the time being. You can't do it all at once unless you don't mind a major time commitment.

If pressed for time, stretch 10 to 15 minutes daily.

Don't forget, you are simply not allowed to stretch cold. It's forbidden!

Stretching first thing in the morning as an expression of wellness is one of the big myths about exercise. For your musculoskeletal frame, it's one of the worst things you can possibly do. The collagen in the muscle is heat dependent. Collagen is hard and inflexible when the temperature in the muscle is low, and it becomes flexible with increased temperature.

Have you ever wondered why ballet dancers tend to wrap themselves in layers and layers of tights and leg warmers? It wasn't just a fashion slip of the 1980s but a smart strategy of increasing the temperature in the muscle.

When you get out of bed in the morning, your muscles are cold. If you stretch before you get up, you will hear the joints cracking loudly in protest. Cracking is feedback that the ligaments were too tight. Cracking your joints repeatedly over time causes arthritis.

Stretching is not a warm-up. Stretching is safe and productive only *after* a warm-up.

If you still want to stretch early in the morning, warm up first. Move all of your limbs for 10 to 15 minutes until you feel your body temperature increase. Increased blood flow in the muscles increases cellular metabolism and temperature, which in turn warms up the collagen.

The best time for stretching is after exercise. Stretching is the ideal cool-down phase after any workout. It prevents muscles from becoming tight after weight lifting, and you'll make the greatest gains in increasing your range of motion while muscular blood flow peaks. You'll be surprised how easily you'll stretch after an hour of exercise. If you haven't exercised and stretched thoroughly for a while or even years, try it and you'll be more comfortable in your own skin.

And no, muscles don't shorten from building muscle. Let's kill this myth before it emerges. If you think about it, muscles attach from one bone across a joint to another bone. The muscles can't shorten, because the bones don't shorten either. What can shorten is the range of motion across the joint, which is caused by inflexibility of muscles and ligaments. If you stretch, you don't need to worry about it. If you don't stretch, you'll get stiff whether you lift weights or not.

Weight lifting doesn't deserve the bad reputation of shortening muscle. Come to think of it, cardiovascular training can make you awfully stiff. Hours of running or bicycling tighten your lower back and hamstrings, which typically causes back pain over time. Have you ever woken up stiff as a brick after a long walk at the beach the day before? Stretching is equally important after any endurance exercise, which includes walking.

The must-stretch-or-else muscles are the back and hamstring muscles, and the hip flexors. These muscles maintain the flexibility of your core because all of them attach to the pelvis. The core is your center of gravity and the origin of all movement, because movement is balanced at your point of gravity.

Let's go over a few basic stretches for this critical area. You may have a thorough repertoire of stretches already and if your stretches address back, hamstrings and hip flexors, by all means keep to your routine. As long as it works and you're stretching every day or every other day, you're covered.

If you're not satisfied with what you know, see the practical instruction section on stretching for easy but effective stretches.

CHAPTER 4

NUTRITION: NEGOTIATING WITH THE ENEMY

Diet and nutrition are touchy subjects. A debate on eating healthy can easily turn as emotional as a discussion about politics or religion. Don't bring it up at a party. Hopefully, your closest friends agree with your philosophy on eating, or it's war. In Los Angeles, you can barely invite friends for dinner unless you arrange for their specialized diet plan. Is it organic, dairy free, sugar free, soy free, low-carb, gluten free, vegan, raw, salt free or sea salt friendly? When it comes to food in Los Angeles, one might think general anxiety is projected onto edibles. As Angelenos, we curb our anxiety by telling ourselves that if we eat right, we can ward off death as though it's a disease caused by poor choices. The (anxiety based) obsession with healthy eating can even progress into a mental disorder, called orthorexia nervosa

Don't argue against someone's survival strategy. It's a battle you can't win. There are plenty of opinions available. If you find the right one that guarantees eternal healthy life, please email me.

This is not to say that you shouldn't strive to eat a healthy diet. Of course you should. Your diet determines your weight, affects your health, and influences your sense of well-being. Educate yourself according to your personal philosophy, pay attention to the effect of food on your system, and optimize what works for you.

My advice is, don't listen to anyone who isn't a licensed professional. If you want to change your diet, choose between a nutritionist or health practitioner, decide between established medicine and a holistic approach, consult with your doctor and come up with a science-based strategy. Read about diet or diet plans, but make sure the books are written by someone with appropriate credentials.

I've seen great results with blood-type or genetic-origin diets, crafted by professionals and based on blood or genetic tests. Diet is not "one size fits all."

Some vegetarians are overweight from overeating carbohydrates. Vegans are frequently anemic. I've seen health-crazed clients go into shock when their blood tests come back with reports of malnourishment. Cutting out entire food groups can be harmful if you don't know what you're doing.

If you want to eat a healthy diet, make sure it's healthy.

IS YOUR DIET HABITUAL OR EMOTIONAL?

I've found that for most women, a lack of nutritional guidance was not the issue. We usually know what to eat and what we shouldn't be eating. If we do it anyway, we are looking at various degrees of food addiction, or the addiction to the pleasure food provides.

Only you can judge where you fit on that scale of mild to moderate or severe. But if emotional eating is the issue and you can't stick to a reasonable weight loss plan, you might consider exploring the causes with a licensed psychotherapist who has experience with emotional eating.

Don't beat yourself up if this is the case. If you pinpoint a problem, it's great news! You have the opportunity to discover what's really missing in your life. You can explore your beliefs about why you think you can't have it, and why you've turned to food as a substitute.

Any unresolved issue you may discover carries within it the opportunity to have what you truly desire.

Let's look at the difference in more detail.

Habits are relatively easy to change. Emotional attachments are not. The two require guidance by very different health professionals.

If weight gains are caused by inactivity, exercise is the way to fix it. If your calorie intake is habitually too high, you can get nutritional guidance and change it. If you can't stick to a nutritional plan, your eating is emotional.

Emotional eating can be imparted in social rituals, such as shared family dinners. Social eating is easier to change than emotional eating. You find that you have a mild attachment to eating with family members, but you're able to stick to a diet plan if you apply self-discipline.

If eating is emotional, food is an important source of relaxation and self-nurturance. You have difficulty maintaining dietary change. You might feel deprived and eventually furious if your favorite foods are crossed off your dietary list. Or you may feel irritable if you're used to the sedation of carbohydrate overkill and you can't relax when you limit your portions. You may use food as a reward, as a safety blanket or comfort.

More often than not, eating is highly emotional, and nutritional advice alone doesn't solve the problem.

You know what you should be doing, but you can't do it. Or you can do it for a while until stress sets in, but during stress you rebel against your self-imposed diet restrictions. Whenever you have an emotional reaction to dietary change, seeking solutions through diet and exercise is pointless. It's not where the real issue is. Unless you address the issue at its source, change is not sustainable.

If food is a non-negotiable source of emotional nurturance, it means you've replaced a mental, emotional, or social need with food. The main purpose of eating is nutritional intake. If food has a highly emotional value for you, you're looking at an opportunity to discover which need of yours has gone unmet.

When you meet your needs satisfactorily, you no longer feel driven to replace satisfaction with food. You'll experience greater life quality and dietary change becomes a breeze.

This is not to say that using food as a reward or finding pleasure in culinary arts is necessarily a sign of psychological imbalance. We all eat foods for pleasure. However, pleasure has a different quality than emotional eating, which is more similar to addiction. Pleasure can be delayed or temporarily replaced. Addiction can't.

If you suspect that your eating is emotional, try working with a licensed mental health professional. Identifying and addressing the root cause of emotional eating can be a valuable opportunity for realignment in the places where you've gone off-course in life. Food can be a drug. Don't settle for short-changing yourself.

SUPERVISED DIET PROGRAMS

If you need to shed a significant amount of weight but watching what you eat combined with exercise doesn't fix the problem, you may need to enroll in a supervised diet program. There are many licensed diet programs and you can also get medical supervision by a specialized doctor, or a bariatrician. You can choose between established or Western medicine, or a holistically oriented doctor.

Some of my clients have been successful with reading books about prescribed diet programs and implementing the suggested strategies, yet the majority achieved best results when enrolled in a program.

Whatever you do, beware of crash diets.

Crash diets are short-term plans of extreme food deprivation, usually found weekly in women's magazines. Crash diets are not endorsed by health care professionals and are not licensed diet programs. They can be exceptionally harmful to your health. I've seen several cases of clients who insisted on crash diets until their malnourishment caused severe symptoms. I've even heard of deaths through diet, even though the underlying issue may have been an eating disorder.

Crash diets rarely work long-term. Sudden food deprivation triggers starvation mode and causes the metabolism to slow down. Once you return to your previous caloric intake, any excess calories will be stored as fat.

The promise of fast weight loss is an unbeatable sales gimmick. Don't fall for fads. Crash diets lower metabolism, often lead to multiple attempts called yo-yo dieting, and typically increase your weight over time.

HEADS UP ON SPORTS NUTRITION

Here's a very short, very basic checklist on sports nutrition. Only a licensed nutritionist or health coach can prescribe an individualized diet plan. The same applies to sports nutrition, and I suggest you find professionals you can trust.

When lifting weights, your goal is building lean muscle mass. Muscles need protein to grow.

Protein consists of 10 essential and 10 non-essential amino acids. It doesn't matter when you consume your daily protein intake as long as the amount is appropriate for your current needs.

A sedentary person needs approximately 0.8 grams per kilo of body weight. An active adult needs 1.2 to 1.5 grams per kilo. Athletes may need more due to increased strain. Seniors may need more due to muscular loss.

If you are lifting weights, 1.5 grams per kilo is a good guideline. Divide your body weight in pounds by 2.2, which is your weight in kilos. Then multiply the amount by 1.5 grams. This is how much protein you need.

Adding a protein powder to your diet can make it much easier to take in all essential and non-essential amino acids. Protein powders mixed with yoghurt, almond milk, or fruit can make a good meal replacement, and it's also much easier to estimate how much protein you have taken in.

Choose your protein powder as carefully as any supplement. Supplements are not regulated by the FDA. There is no guarantee the label keeps its promise. Some vitamin supplements or protein powders have shown traces of heavy metals in lab tests. Buy only from trusted companies.

Eggs are the most high quality source of protein you can get. Soy has been said to mimic estrogen in the body and some nutritionists caution to stay away from it. Whey is a good choice for optimal muscle recovery; the protein is derived from dairy. Get sound advice from a professional who shares your personal food philosophy.

Good hydration is essential during exercise, but even more so during weight loss.

The guidelines for water intake vary, depending on food philosophy. The most common suggestion is drinking 64 ounces of water per day, but water intake is better adjusted to body weight, climate, and activity levels.

Water intake influences fat loss. Since the liver is needed to break down fat, liver function must be optimized. When the kidneys are under-functioning due to a lack of fluids in the system, the liver will engage in the detoxifying process. A busy liver is not an effective liver. Flush the kidneys so the liver can break down fat. Urine should be colorless. If it isn't, you're dehydrated.

Include antioxidants in your diet. Choose fruit and vegetables over supplements. The body can tell the difference, since the real thing has additional phytonutrients not found in pills.

Exercise increases oxygen consumption, which in turn increases the production of free radicals. Yes, breathing is actually harmful. Since we can't do without it and increased oxygen consumption has more benefits than downfalls, amp up your daily antioxidants.

DIETING AIDS

Stay away from diet pills. Supplements are not FDA regulated. If it wasn't prescribed by a trusted physician, you don't know what you're taking. Some over-the-counter diet pills are so harmful it's hard to believe they are still legal. If you use them anyway, look up the ingredients on the back of the package and conduct thorough research on what they are and what they do. You might toss the bottle in horror. Bariatric or holistic doctors may prescribe safe diet pills, but typically only after taking a blood test.

If you're struggling with food cravings or ravenous hunger

attacks, you may be on an insulin rollercoaster. High levels of insulin and resulting low blood sugar is the most common cause for why women turn to diet pills, because the food cravings caused by low blood sugar are so hard to resist.

Try excluding refined sugar from your diet and reduce carbohydrate intake. Withdrawing sugar from your system lowers insulin levels, which in turn lowers food cravings. Try replacing carbohydrates with protein, as protein doesn't trigger high levels of insulin.

When refined sugar or carbohydrates are broken down and enter the bloodstream as energy, the pancreas releases insulin. Insulin is needed to utilize the circulating energy and make it available to the cells.

A high amount of sugars requires a high amount of insulin. While sugars are necessary energy for cell metabolism, sugars also provide short-term energy. In other words, the energy wasn't meant to last. Once insulin distributes sugars into the cells, blood sugar levels drop. Low blood sugar causes ravenous hunger.

The higher your carbohydrate intake, the more dramatic the blood sugar drops. You'll be ravenous every few hours and dieting can seem like torture.

Withdrawing refined sugar and limiting carbohydrate intake can feel like drug withdrawal for four to six days. After a week, your system adjusts to lower insulin production and the hunger pangs will subside.

A diet high in protein and vegetables does not cause high levels of insulin, and you'll find yourself needing far less food because you're less hungry.

Since any dietary adjustment must fit your personal needs, reducing carbohydrate intake is most safely done with the help of a health professional. Increasing protein intake is usually safe, but can be problematic for individuals prone to developing kidney stones.

PART 3: PRACTICAL INSTRUCTION

Chapter 1

THE BASIC WORKOUT

The Basic Workout is a blue print for any complete weight lifting routine. It shows you one to two exercises for each of the major muscle groups, and it gives examples of the most common mistakes that lead to injury or discomfort.

For each muscle group, you can plug in different exercises including machines and freeweights. You can add exercises for upper or lower body as long as you work agonist and antagonist equally. For example, if you want to add exercises for the legs, you add equally to the quadriceps and hamstring group. If you add exercises for the thigh, you add equally to inner and outer thigh.

The nine major muscle groups should be worked two to three times per week, with 48 hours of rest in between workouts.

Every advanced workout is only a variation of the Basic Workout. Using the Basic Workout as a blue print ensures developing the entire body and avoiding muscular imbalances that can lead to injuries.

1) THE CORE

1. ABDOMINALS (RECTUS ABDOMINIS)

Working abdominal muscles correctly is the most difficult exercise to learn, so give yourself some time and be very mindful to get it right. The difficulty is in engaging the abdominal muscles without using additional upper body muscles.

We are natural cheaters when it comes to physical exertion. Straining one muscle group while relaxing all the others goes against survival instinct. If you overly strain one muscle, you could injure it and be unable to run away from predators. Unless you recondition yourself consciously, you will take the strain off the muscle once it begins to work hard and utilize other muscle groups. However, we want to isolate muscles and strain them just right so they will grow. It takes practice and skill, so you need to listen to your body and engage every muscle group consciously.

If you're a beginner, I suggest you start with equipment to build the abdominals. Most gyms have abdominal rollers, abdominal benches, or large gym balls. I will show you abdominal crunches using a gym ball because most gyms have them. Once you understand the movement, you can apply it to a different piece of equipment.

For your advanced cycles, I will also show you abdominal crunches on the floor. It's the most common and well-known abdominal exercise. You lie on your back with bent knees, keep your hands folded behind the neck, and pull the upper body off the floor.

You can always perform abdominal crunches on the mat when you don't have access to equipment. But mat crunches can be difficult if you don't yet have enough strength to lift the upper body off the floor. You may compensate with other muscles, strain your neck and suffer tension headaches after exercise.

Equipment such as abdominal rollers or benches are very helpful for beginners, because you can use the head rest to support the neck until the abdominals are strong enough to lift the upper body off the floor. When you begin with head and neck support to compensate for weak abdominal muscles, it is easier to build the abdominals without straining neck muscles. However, not every gym has such equipment, so I won't feature it here. If you learn how to do abdominal crunches on the ball or floor, you can use any equipment because you will understand the correct movement.

Abdominal crunches require a much higher amount of repetitions, because crunches are not a weight bearing exercise. There are no weights to stack up; you only move the weight of the upper body. It's a low intensity exercise. You increase the intensity by performing more repetitions.

Start with three sets, of 12 to 20 repetitions. Pay careful attention to how many repetitions you can perform before you begin pulling on your neck. When you notice that you are losing correct form, stop. It's the maximum amount of repetitions you can do. Rest for a minute, then do your next set. Aim for the same number of repetitions you did earlier.

Work up to three sets of 20. Increase the sets and repetitions as you get stronger. Aim for building up to eight sets of 50 repetitions, or four sets of 100 repetitions. If you want a beautifully sculpted and strong core, work up to 450 repetitions total for abdominals and obliques combined.

Because core work is of a lower intensity, you can and should exercise it more often than other muscles. Once you can perform crunches safely without equipment, it is good practice to fit in extra sets at home.

If you are uncertain how often you should do abdominal work, listen to your body. If you exercised your core the previous day but you can still perform a number of sets the next, you are in the clear. If the muscles are obviously exhausted and you can't perform the full range of motion, the muscles need rest.

Now, how do you know you're engaging the abdominals? Imagine you're making a fist with your abs when you pull the upper body off the floor. The muscles should stay in a state of tension as if you balled them to a fist. Keep this tension during each set. As you continue throughout the set, you should feel an increasing burning sensation. The burn is what makes a muscle. The more tension you keep, the more muscle you make. Cheating yourself by doing a high number of repetitions but feeling no tension or burn is cheating yourself out of the results. It's not in the numbers, it's in the burn. Only keep up the burn as long as you can maintain correct form.

It's the hardest exercise to do correctly. But when you learn how to do it right, you'll build a beautifully sculpted abdomen, an hourglass waist, and you'll be free of back pain.

A) BEGINNERS: ABDOMINAL CRUNCHES ON THE BALL

Three sets, 12 to 20 repetitions.

Rest 30 to 60 seconds between sets.

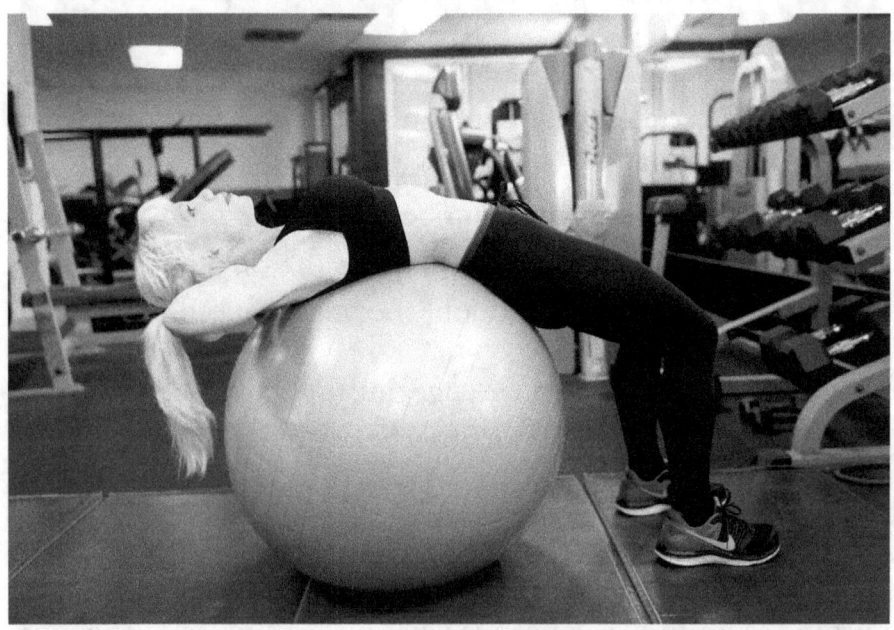

Lie backward over the ball and fold your hands behind your neck. Point your nose to the ceiling. The neck must remain straight and relaxed.

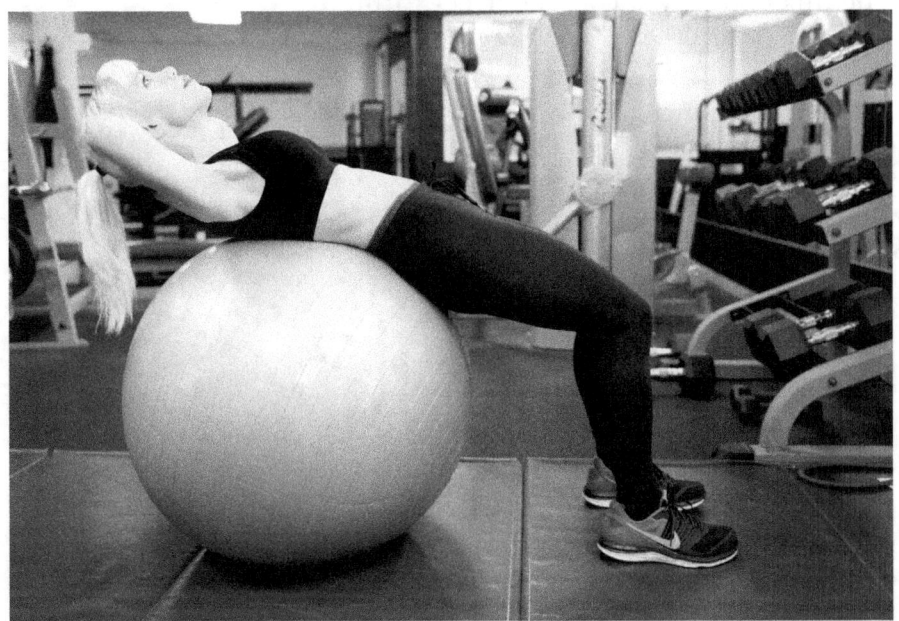

Breathe in before you begin, and then breathe out as you lift the upper body to a 45-degree angle or a nearly straight position. Maintain as much tension in the abdominals as you can.

Breathe in as you return to the starting position. Maintain abdominal tension throughout the entire set.

Count to three as you lift, and count to three as you lower the upper body. Three seconds per movement engages the muscle and prevents using momentum.

The image below shows incorrect form.

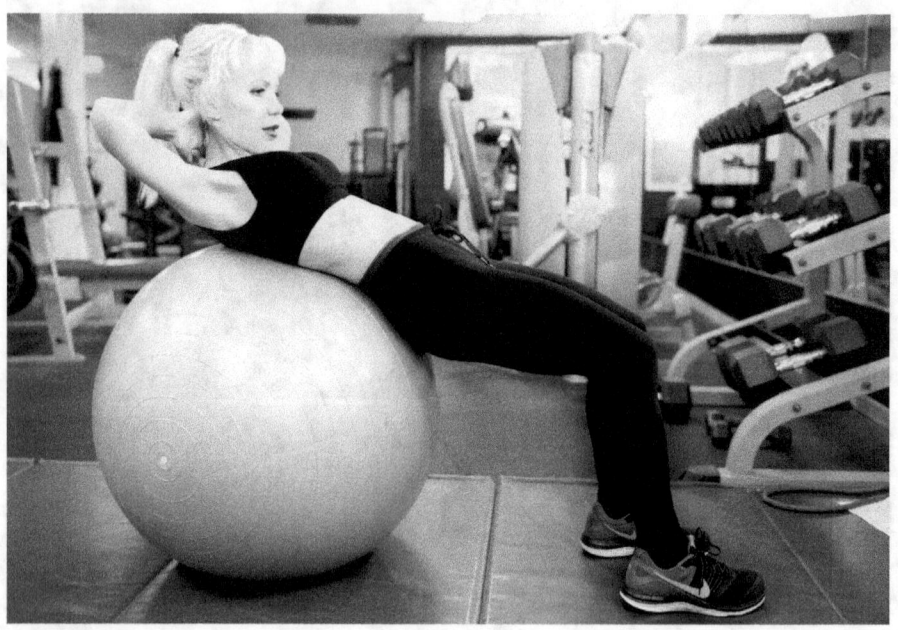

Here, the chin is pulling to the chest, which strains the neck. Common mistakes include using upper body strength and momentum to lift the upper body or lower it. You would feel no or little tension in the abdominals.

B) ADVANCED: ABDOMINAL CRUNCHES ON THE MAT

Three sets, 12 to 20 repetitions.

Lie on your back and fold your hands behind your neck. Point your nose toward the ceiling. The neck must remain straight and relaxed.

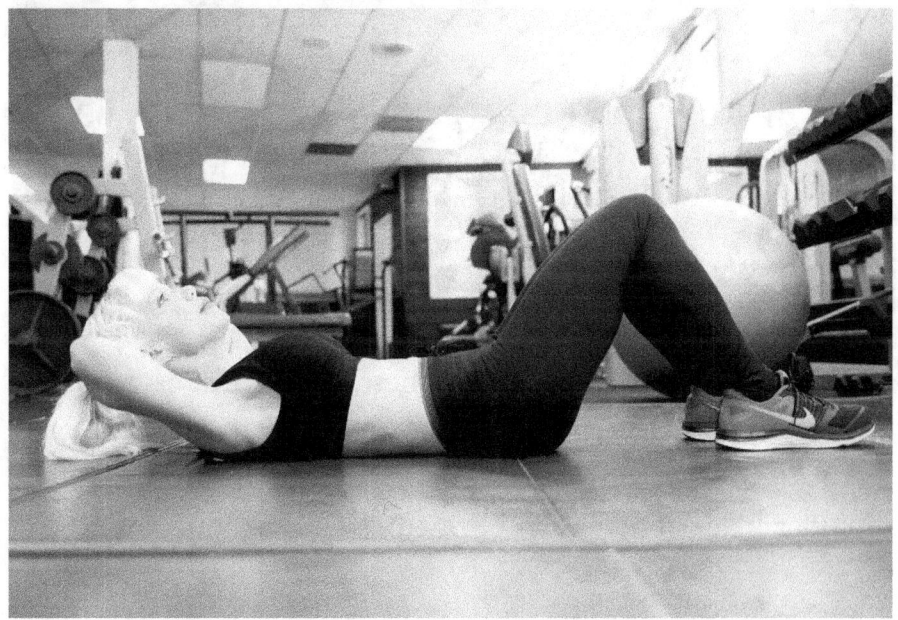

Breathe in before you begin, and then breathe out as you lift the upper body off the floor.

Breathe in as you lower the upper body, but maintain tension in the abdominals. In the lowered position, keep the shoulder blades off the floor. Perform the entire set without allowing the shoulder blades to touch the floor. Count to three as you lift, and count to three as you lower the upper body.

The image below shows incorrect form.

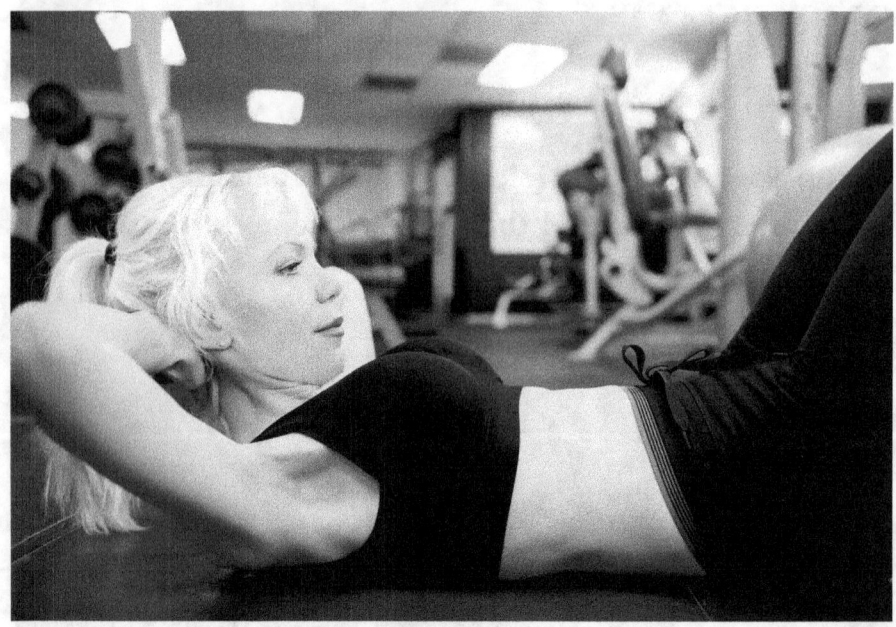

Here, the chin is pulling to the chest, which strains the neck. Common mistakes include using upper body strength and momentum to "swing" the upper body up, and touching the shoulder blades on the floor which relaxes the muscles during the set.

2. OBLIQUES (TRANSVERSE ABDOMINIS)

A) BEGINNERS: STANDING OBLIQUE BENDS

Three sets, 12 to 20 repetitions.

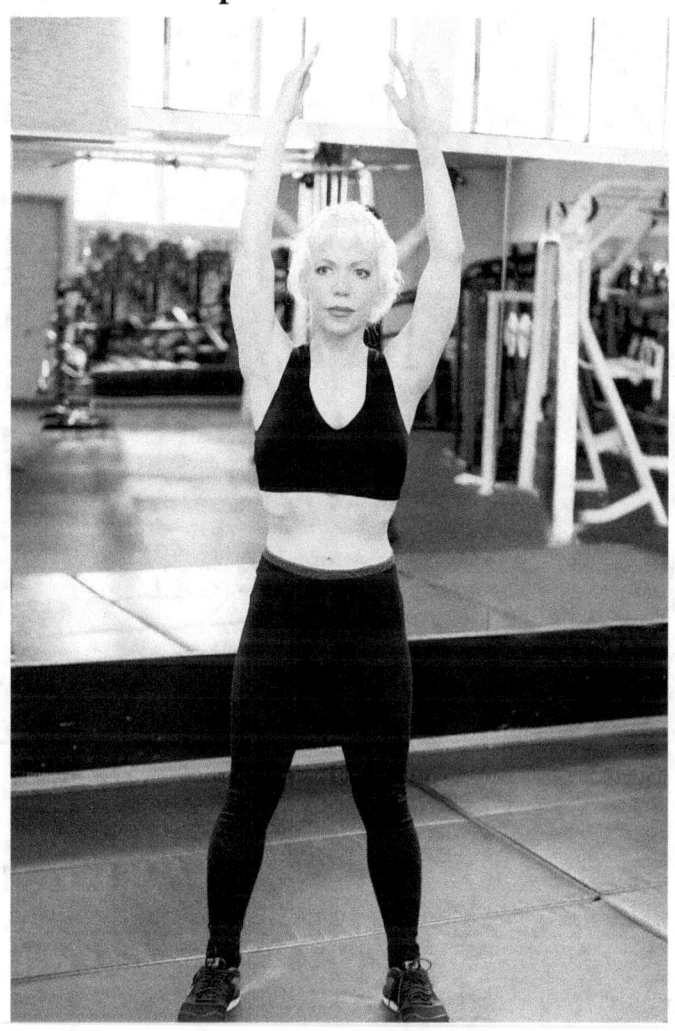

Stand with your legs at shoulder width apart and extend your arms up. Keep the shoulders down to minimize neck tension.

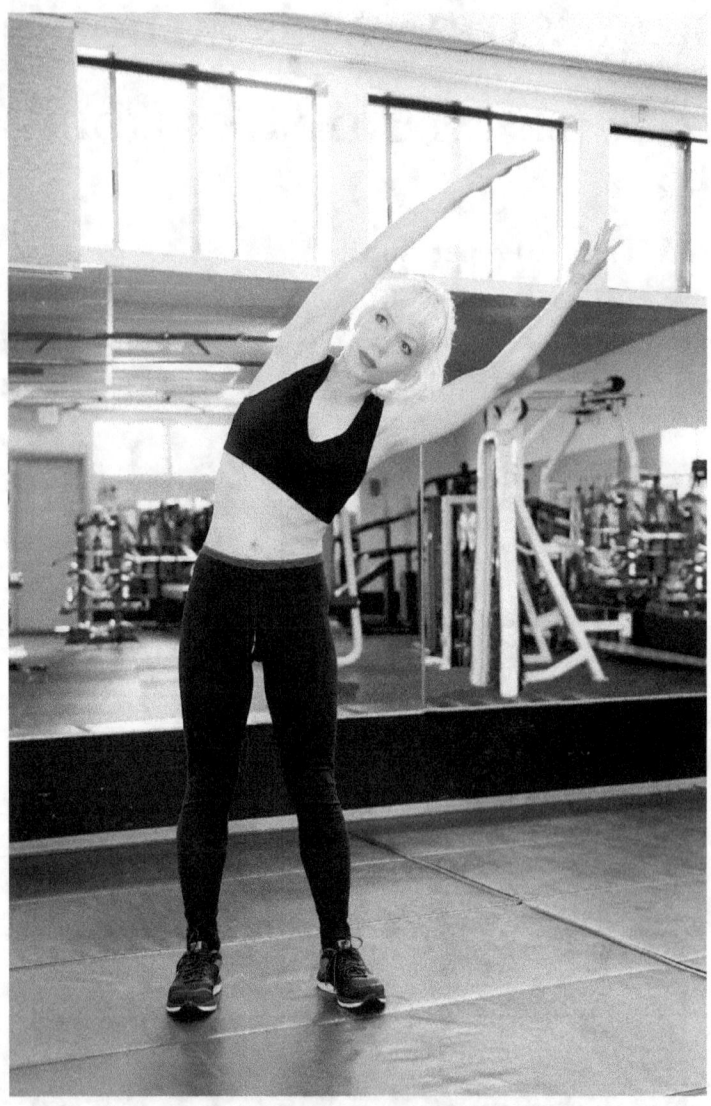

Breathe in as you tilt the upper body. Maintain straight hips. Breathe out as you return to the starting position.

Take turns tilting to the right and to the left.

Count to three as you tilt the upper body, and count to three as you straighten.

The image below shows incorrect form.

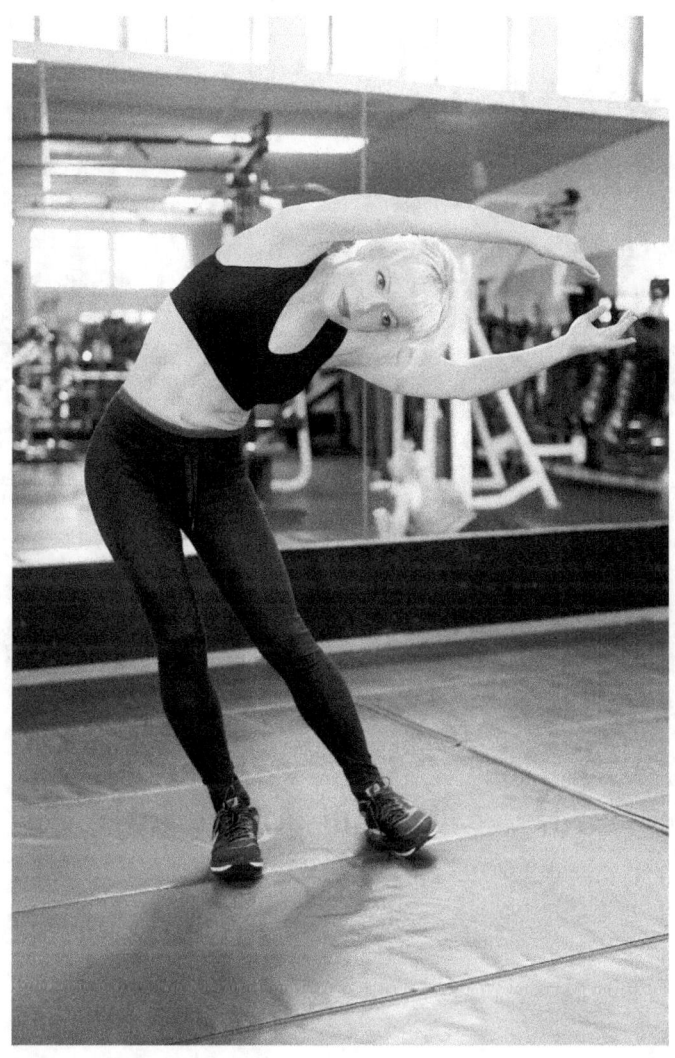

Here, the hips are tilted. I'm exaggerating the mistake so you can see what I mean. The movement is performed by swinging or tilting the entire body. This fails to isolate and engage the oblique muscles at the waist.

B) ADVANCED: OBLIQUES OVER THE BALL

Three sets, 12 to 20 repetitions.

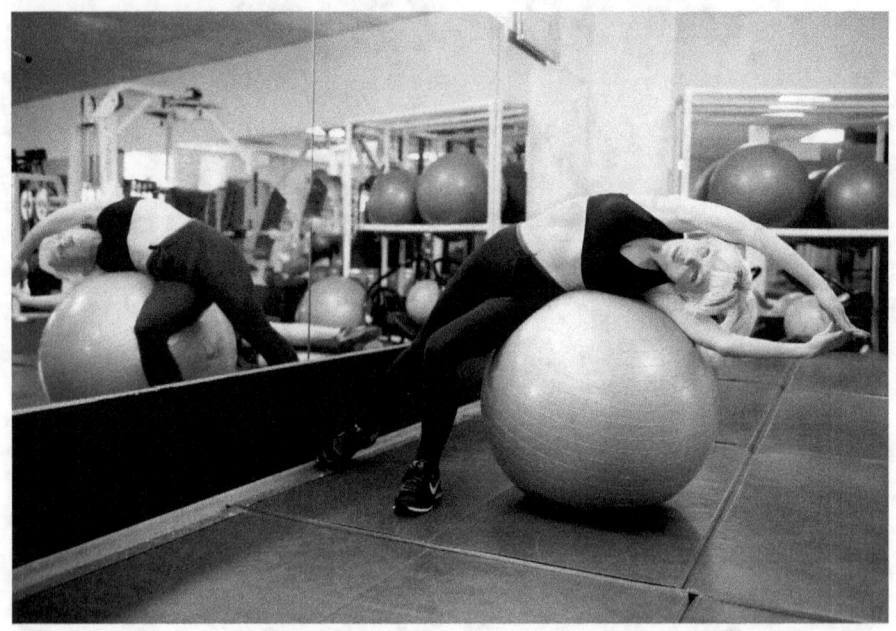

Lay sideways over a ball, stabilizing your feet against a wall. Extend your arms above your head.

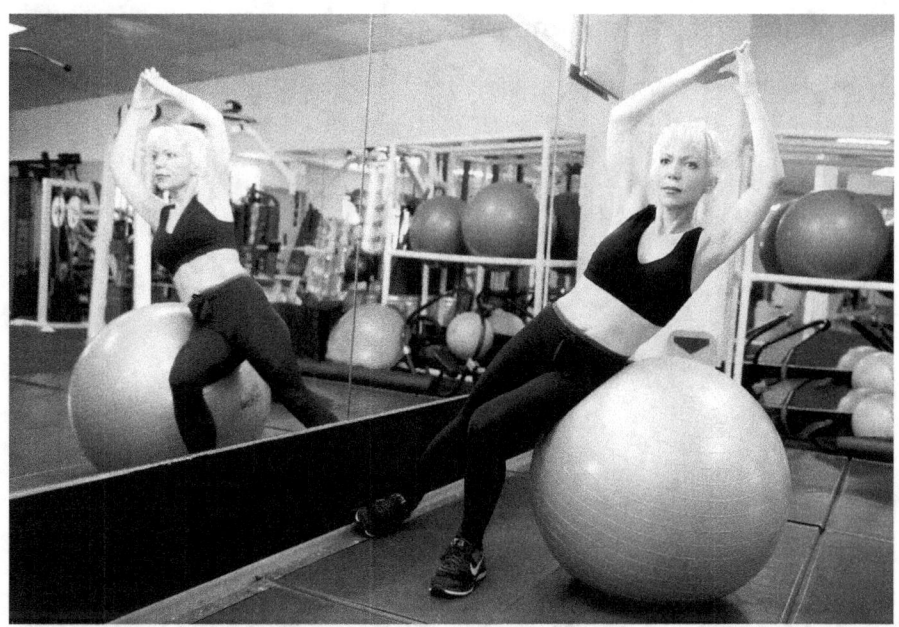

Breathe in before you begin, and then breathe out as you lift the upper body. Breathe in as you return to the starting position.

Count to three as you lift up, and count to three as you lower the upper body.

The image below shows incorrect form.

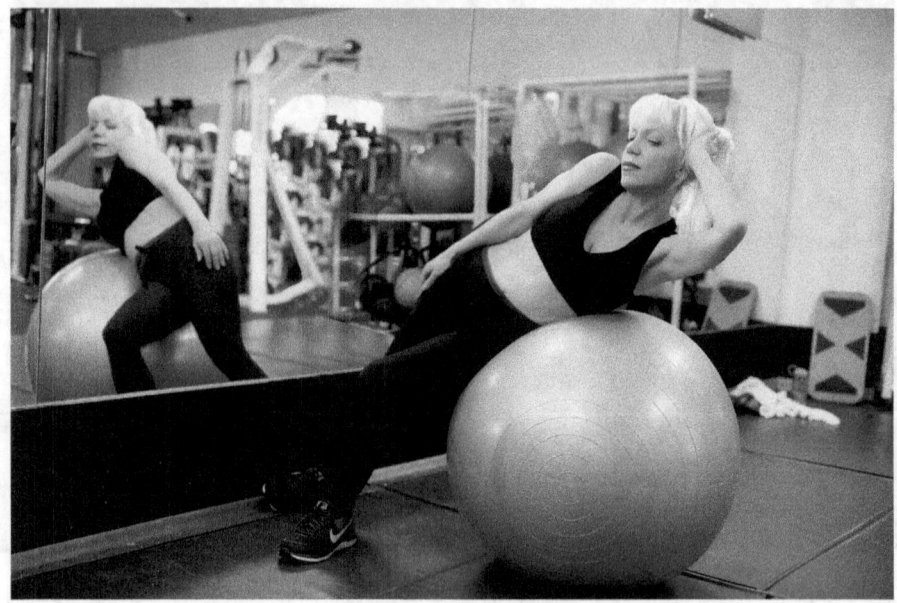

Here, the shoulders are drawn up, straining the upper back and the neck. Instead of bending the waist, the neck is bent. It may feel as if you are bending from the waist, but most of the muscular tension is in the neck and upper back. The range of motion is too small, failing to engage the obliques fully.

3. LOWER BACK (ERECTOR SPINAE)

BACK EXTENSIONS

Three sets, 12 to 20 repetitions.

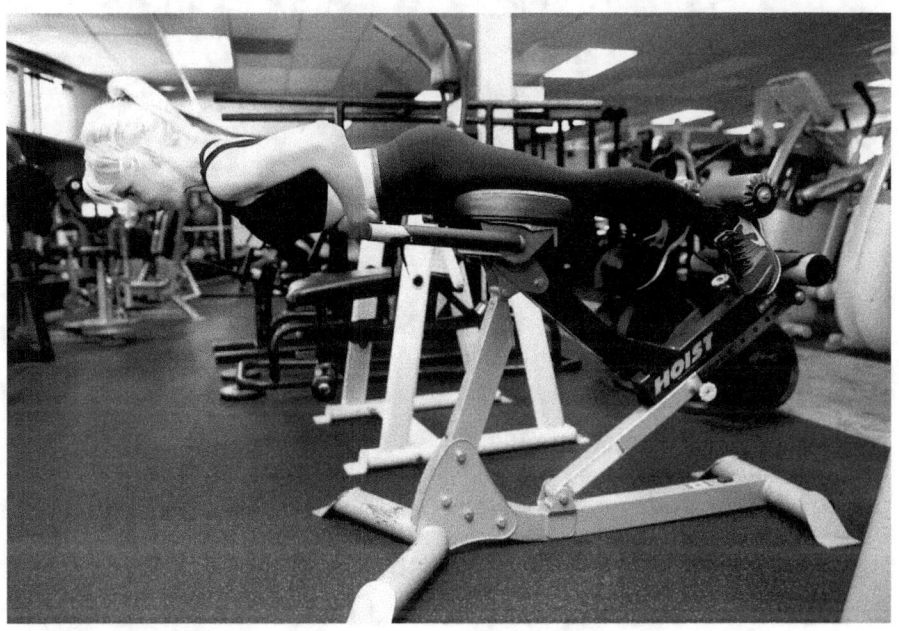

Tuck your feet in safely and extend your body forward in a straight line.

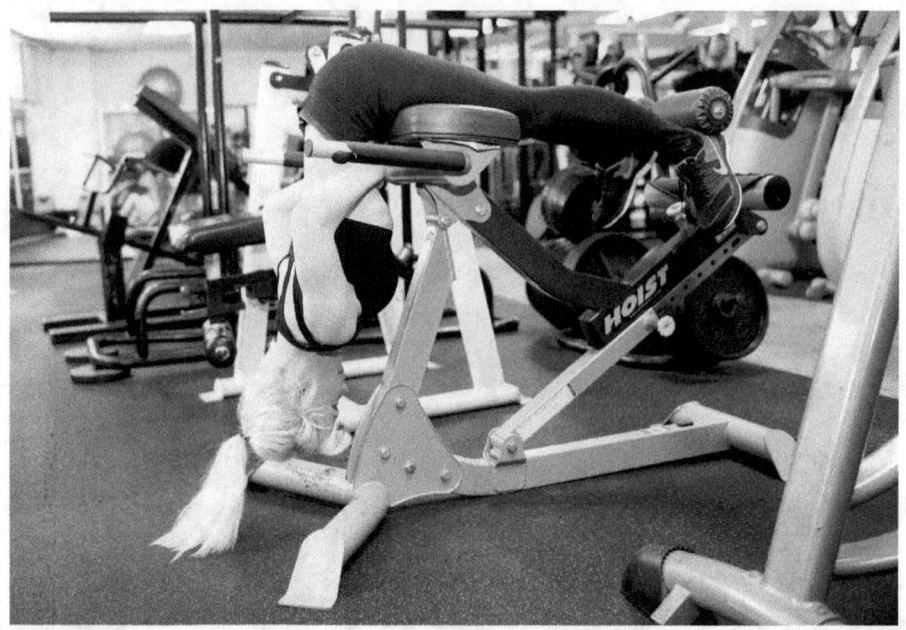

Breathe in as you lower the upper body to a 90° angle in relation to your legs. Pause at the bottom of the exercise to allow for spinal traction.

Breathe out as you return to the starting position. Keep your back straight. Pause at the extended position.

Count to three as you lower the upper body, and count to three as you raise the upper body.

The image below shows incorrect form.

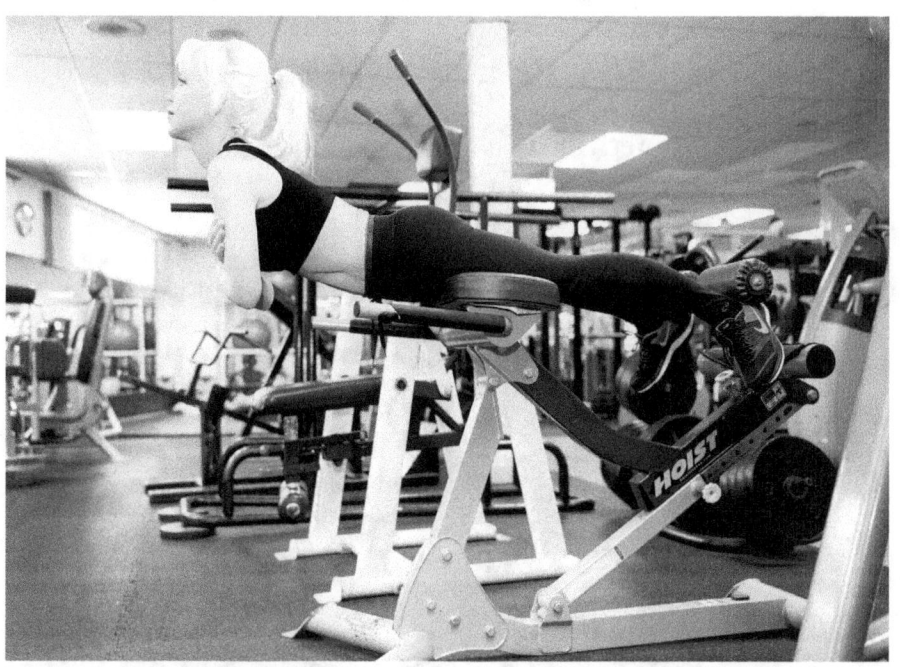

Here, the back is arched. Due to the pull of gravity on your upper body, it can compress lower back discs and lead to discomfort.

2) THE CHEST (PECTORALIS MAJOR)

SEATED CHEST PRESS

Three sets, 12 repetitions.

Rest 30 to 60 seconds between sets.

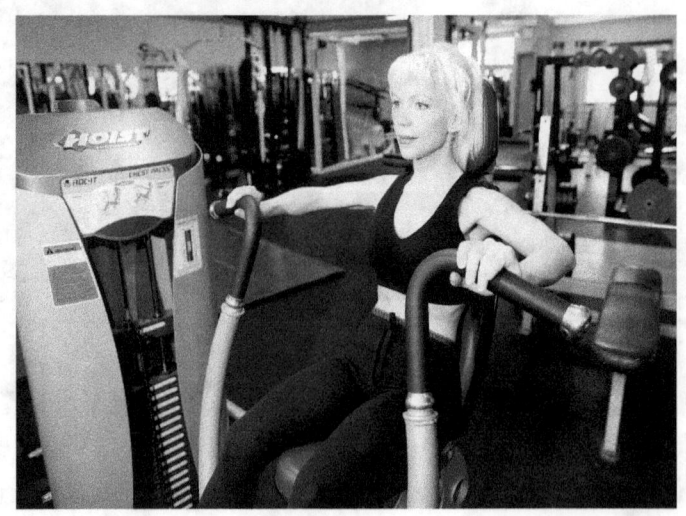

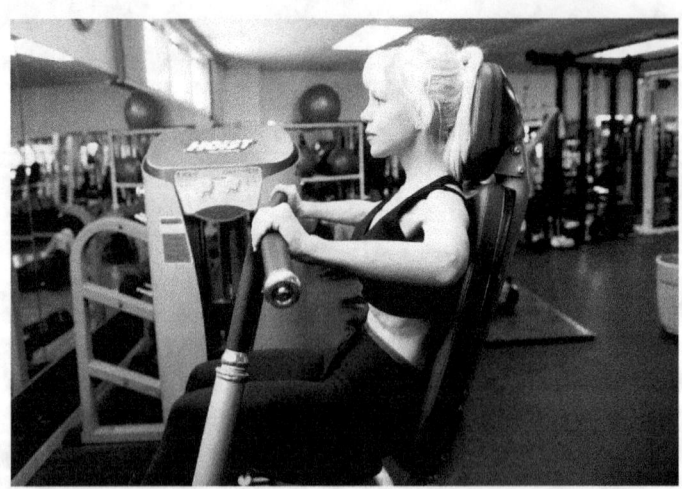

In the starting position, the elbow is aligned with the shoulder.

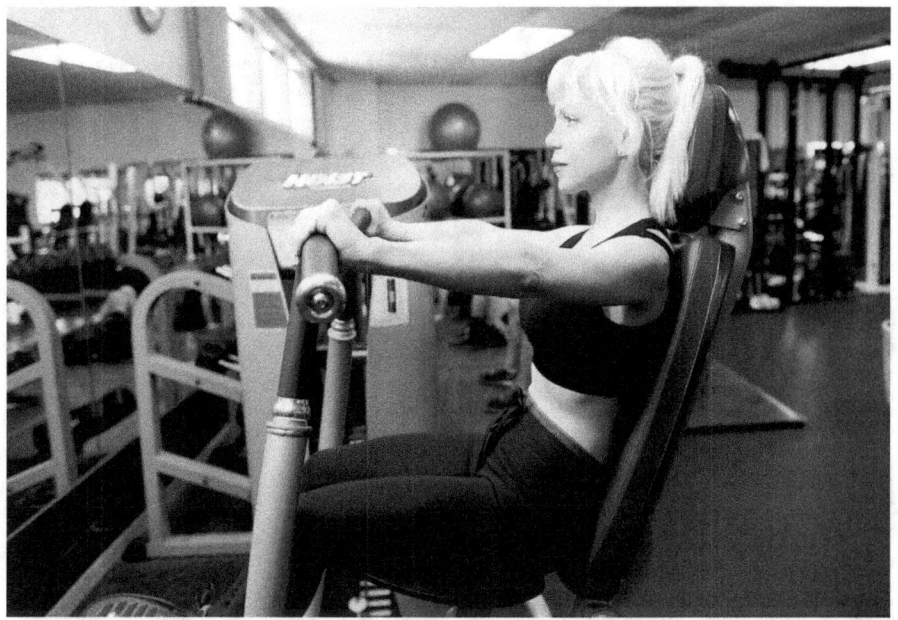

Breathe in first, and then breathe out as you straighten the arms.

Pinch the shoulder blades together and keep your shoulders on the back pad of the machine. Extend your arms fully, but don't lock your elbows.

Breathe in as you return to the starting position.

Imagine your shoulders as a line. Do not bring the elbow farther back than the line of your shoulders. Do not bring the elbows down to the sides of your body.

Count to three as you extend the arms, and count to three as you return to the starting position.

The images below show incorrect form.

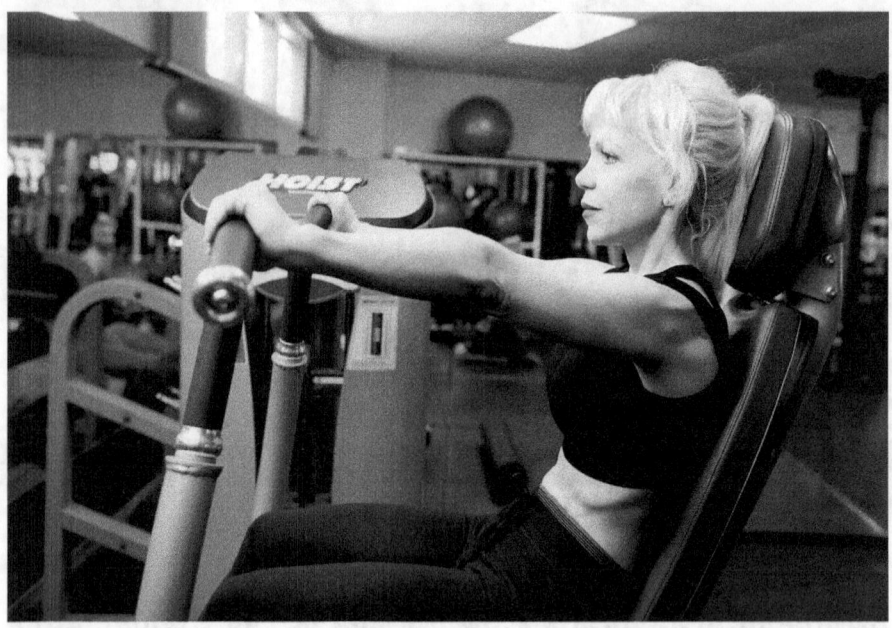

Here, the shoulders are pulled forward and come off the back pad. This puts unnecessary stress on the rotator cuff, and leads to tight upper back muscles which cause tension headaches. Locked elbows damage the joints over time.

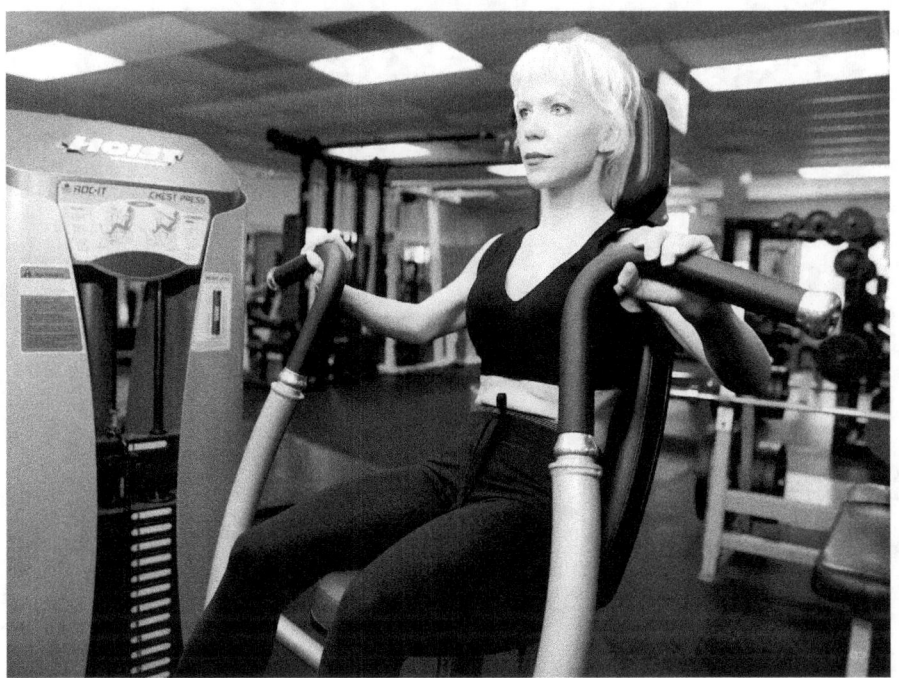

Another common mistake is pulling the elbows close to the body. Lowered elbows take tension off the chest muscle and engage the triceps instead, which fails to develop the target muscle.

3) THE BACK (LATISSIMUS DORSI)

SEATED ROW

Three sets, 12 repetitions.

Rest 30 to 60 seconds between sets.

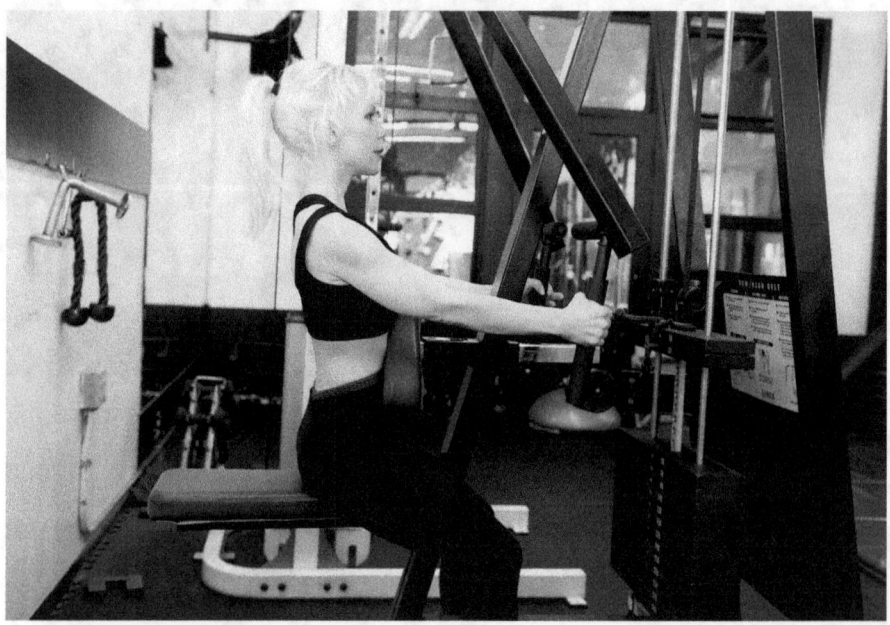

Start by sitting upright with your arms extended in front of you. Be sure the shoulder blades are pinched together, and the shoulders stay down and back. The position shouldn't look any different than when you lift your arms.

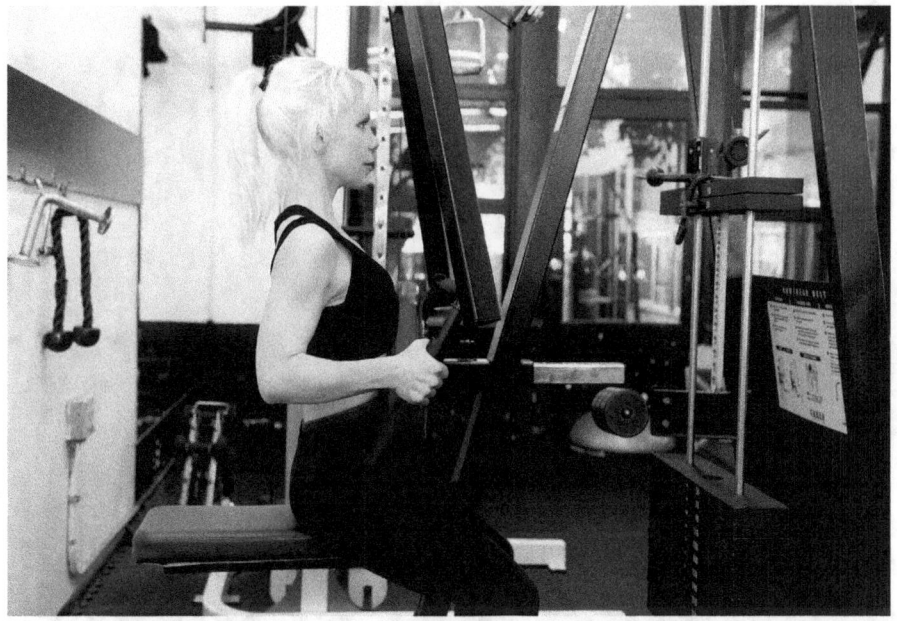

Breathe in, and then breathe out as you pull towards your body. Keep your elbows close to your sides. Don't pull the chin to your chest during the "heavy" phase.

Breathe in as you return to the starting position.

Count to three as you pull, and count to three as you return to the starting position.

The image below shows incorrect form.

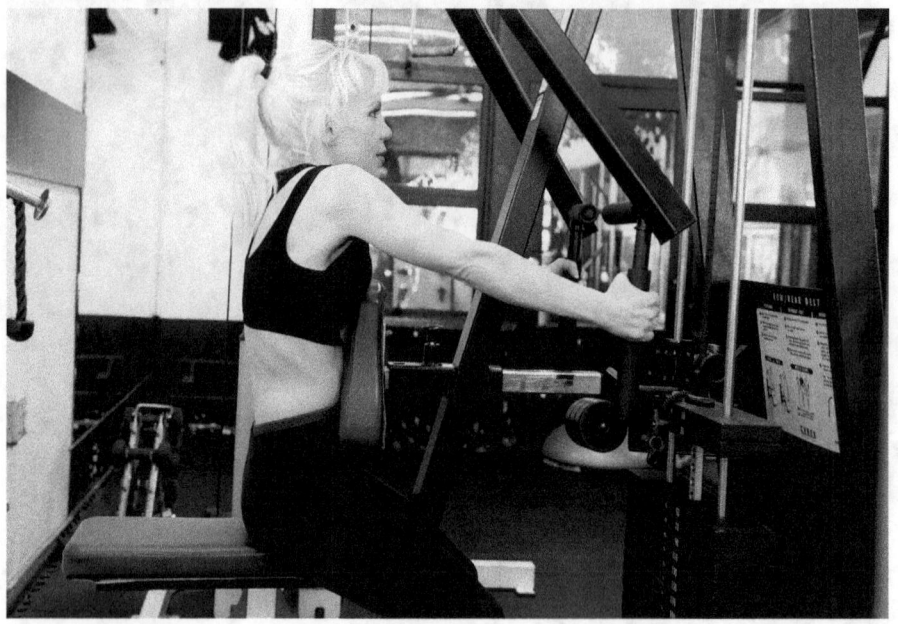

The shoulders are coming forward and up, and the back is rounded. There is tension on the neck, and you may injure the shoulders.

4) THE SHOULDERS (DELTOID)

LATERAL DUMBBELL RAISE

Three sets, 12 repetitions.

Rest 30 to 60 seconds between sets.

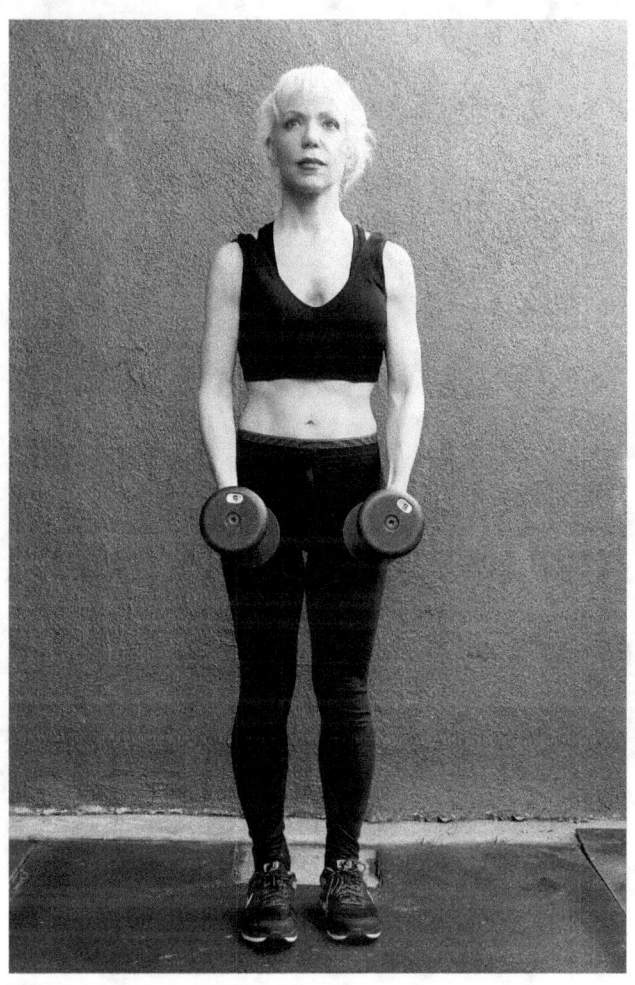

Stand upright and hold the dumbbells in front of you with slightly bent arms. Keep your abs tight—navel pulling to the spine—so that you don't sway backward.

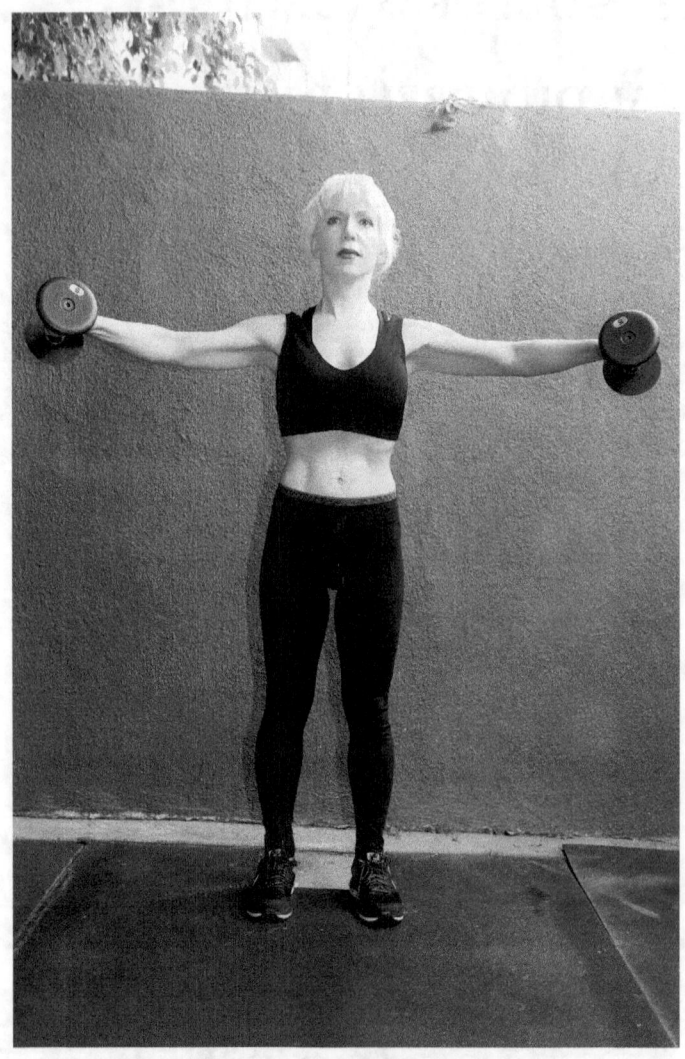

Breathe in first, and then breathe out as you raise the dumbbells to shoulder height. The elbows should be straight but not locked.

Breathe in as you return to the starting position.

Count to three during the lift, and count to three as you return to the starting position.

The image below shows incorrect form.

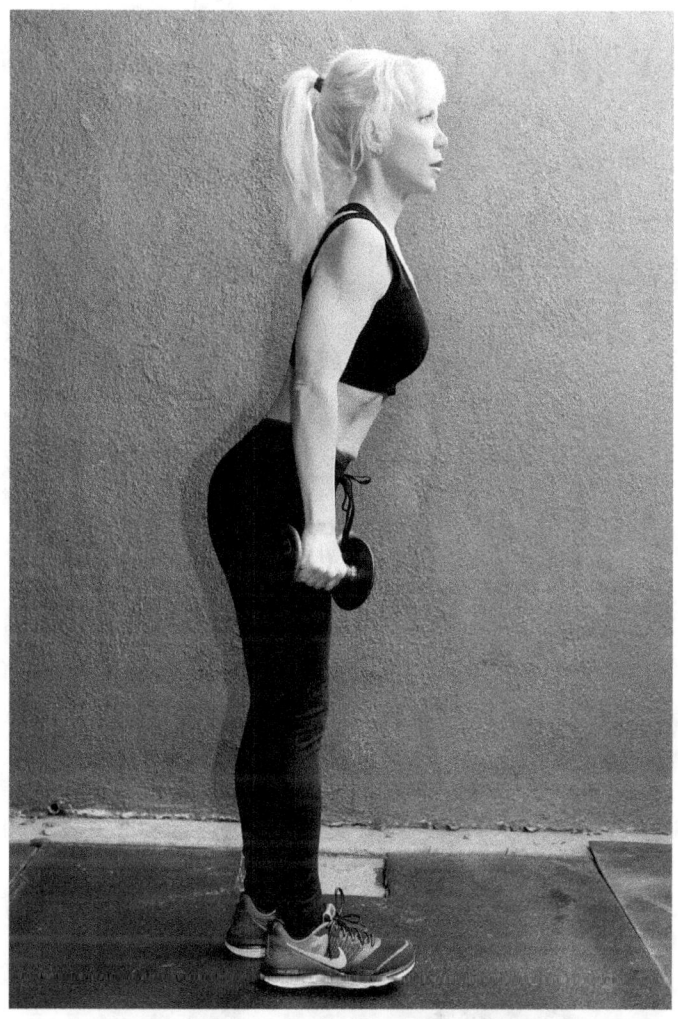

Arching your back and neck while lifting dumbbells compresses discs at the lumbar and cervical spine and can lead to back strain and tension headaches. I'm exaggerating the mistakes grossly so you can see them.

5) THE TRICEPS (TRICEPS BRACHII)

TRICEPS PULL DOWN

Three sets, 12 repetitions.

Rest 30 to 60 seconds between sets.

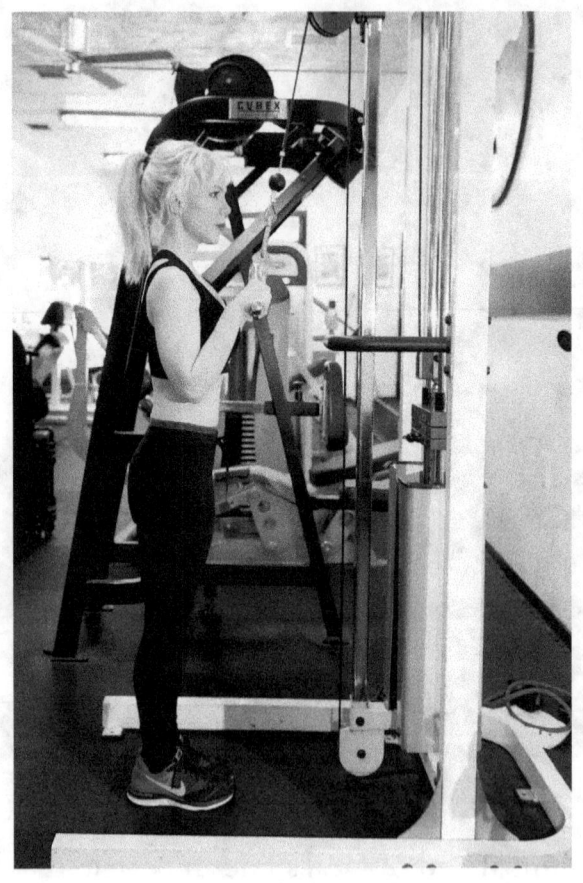

Start by standing upright. Bend your arms as you hold the grip in front of your chest, and tuck your elbows at your sides. The knees should be slightly bent, so you don't lock the joints. Keep the abs tight so your back is straight.

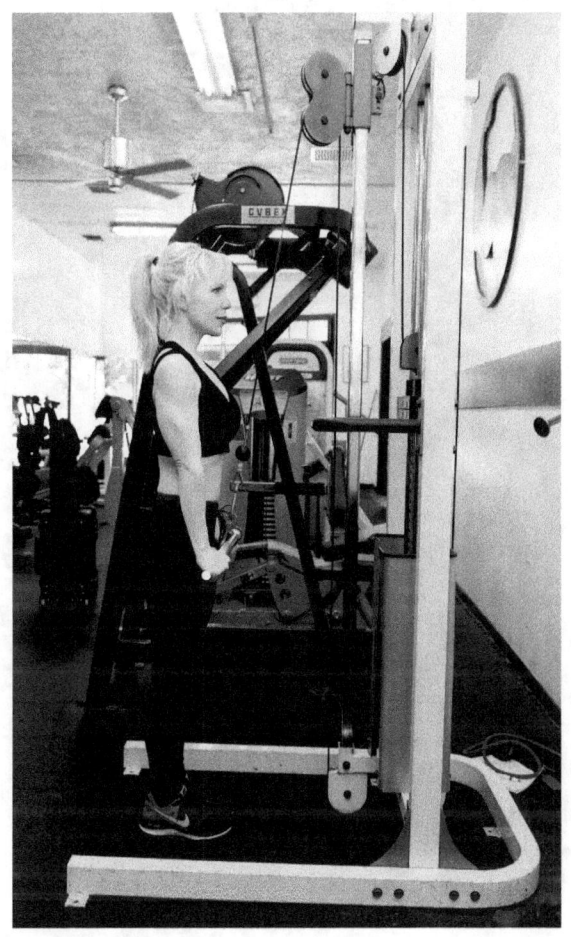

Breathe in, and then breathe out as you extend the arms, pulling the grip toward your thighs. Maintain an upright position.

Breathe in as you return to the starting position.

Count to three as you extend the arms, and count to three as you return to the starting position.

The image below shows incorrect form.

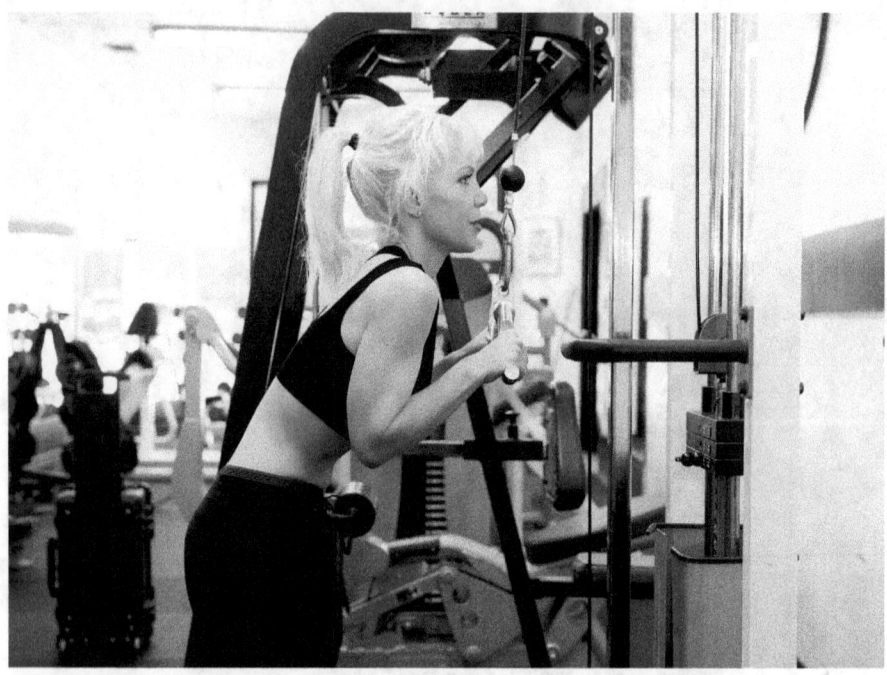

Here, the weight is moved with momentum from the upper body. The shoulders are coming up, which creates neck tension. The triceps is not fully engaged and won't develop.

6) THE BICEPS (BICEPS BRACHII)

BICEPS DUMBBELL CURL

Three sets, 12 repetitions.

Rest 30 to 60 seconds between sets.

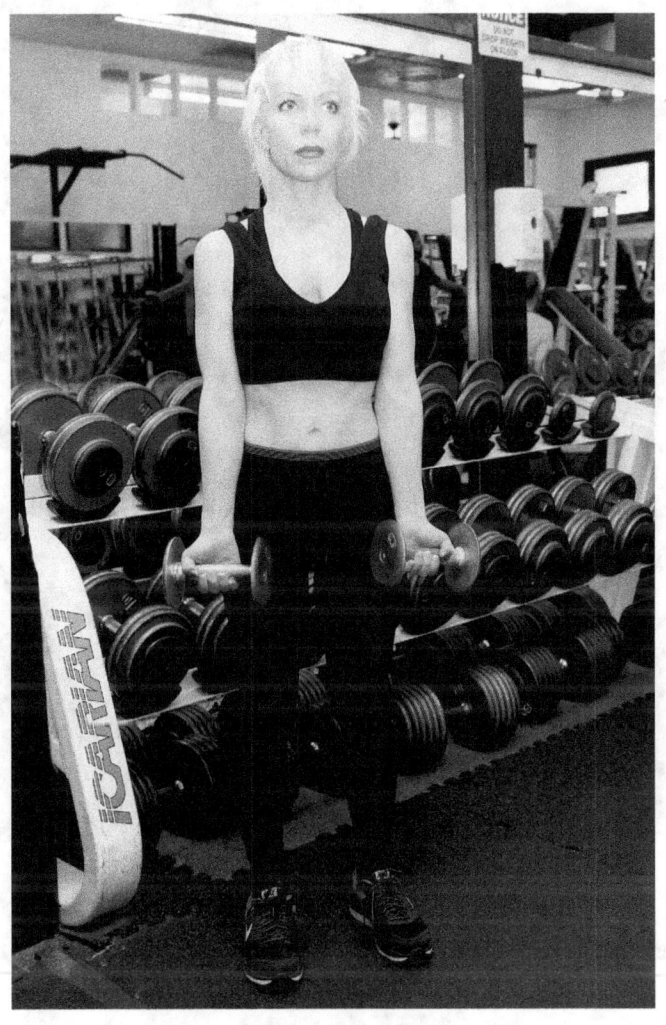

Start by standing upright, holding two dumbbells so they rest on top of your thighs.

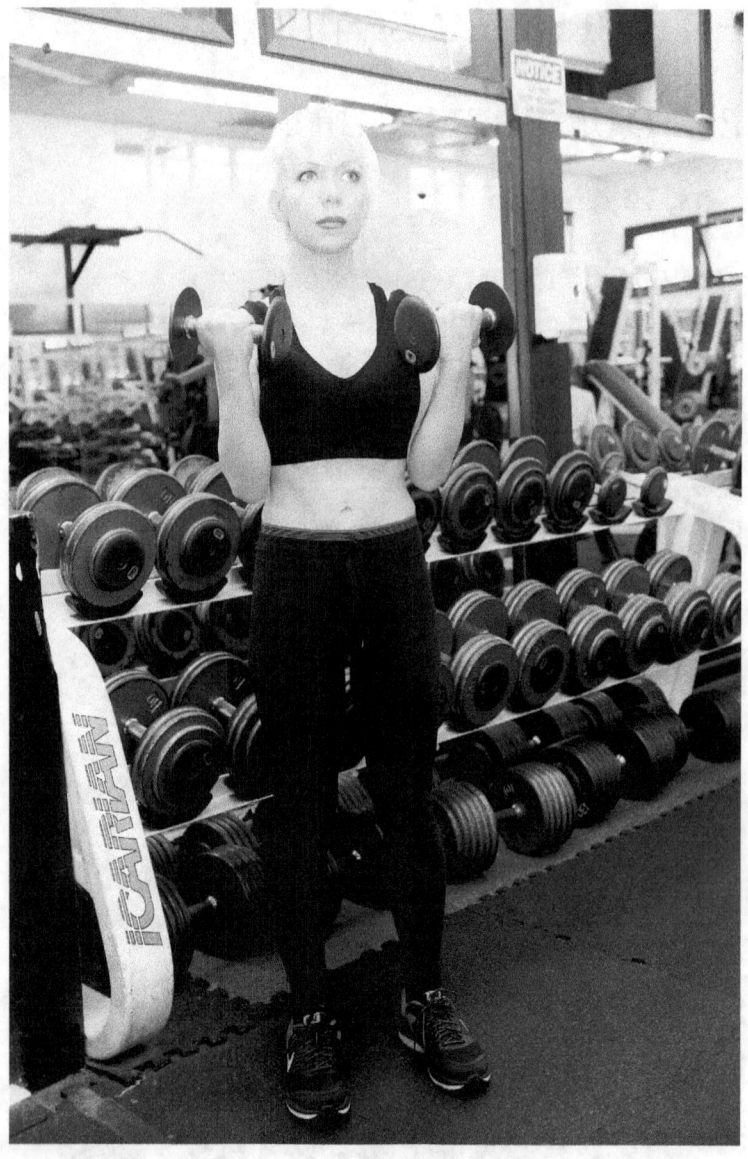

Breathe in first, and then breathe out as you bring the dumbbells toward your chest. Maintain a straight back.

Breathe in as you return to the starting position. Straighten the arm fully at the bottom of the exercise.

Count to three as you bend your arms, and count to three as you straighten.

The image below shows incorrect form.

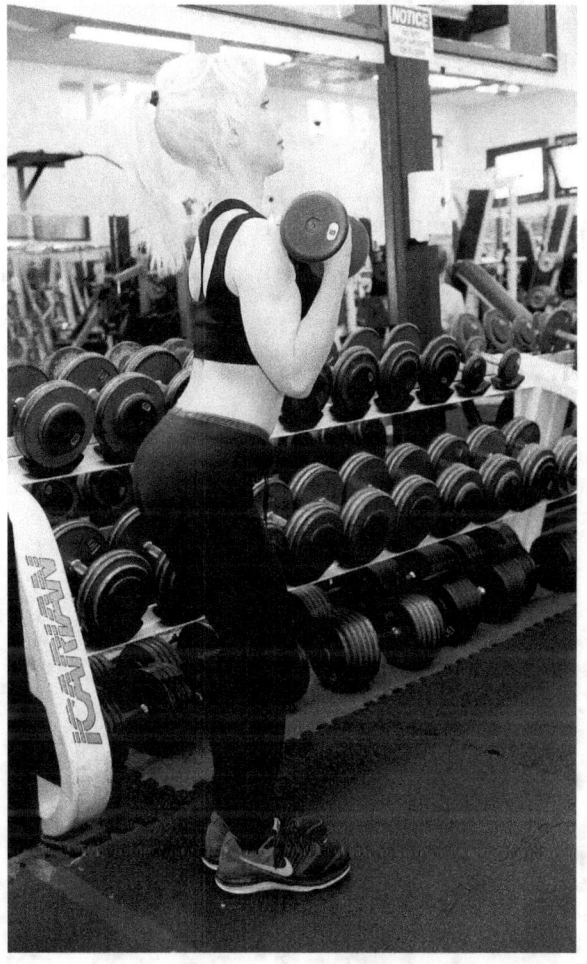

Here, the back is arched during the movement, which can injure the lower back. The mistake is exaggerated for clarity. Additional mistakes include using momentum to "swing" the dumbbells upwards or down, which doesn't engage the muscle fully.

7) THE QUADRICEPS (QUADRICEPS FEMORIS)

LEG EXTENSIONS

Three sets, 12 repetitions.

Rest 30 to 60 seconds between sets.

On this machine it is important to adjust the seat correctly. The knees should be in alignment with the foot lever. The foot lever is pulled upward during leg extensions. If the knees are sticking out farther than the foot lever of the machine, there will be stress on the knees.

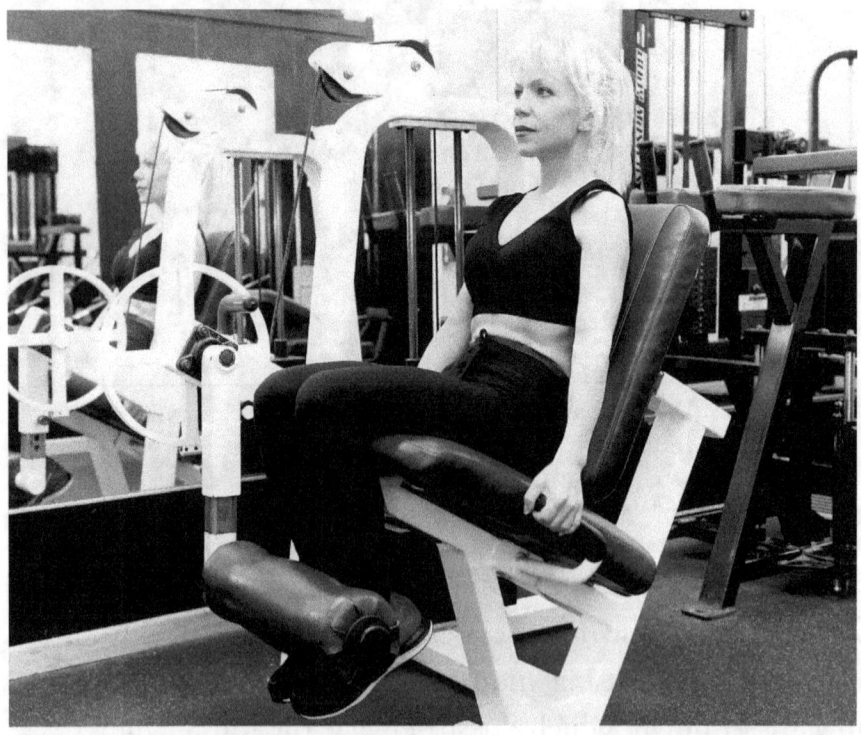

Start with the legs bent. Use the grips on both sides of the

seat, so your pelvis doesn't move up as you straighten your legs.

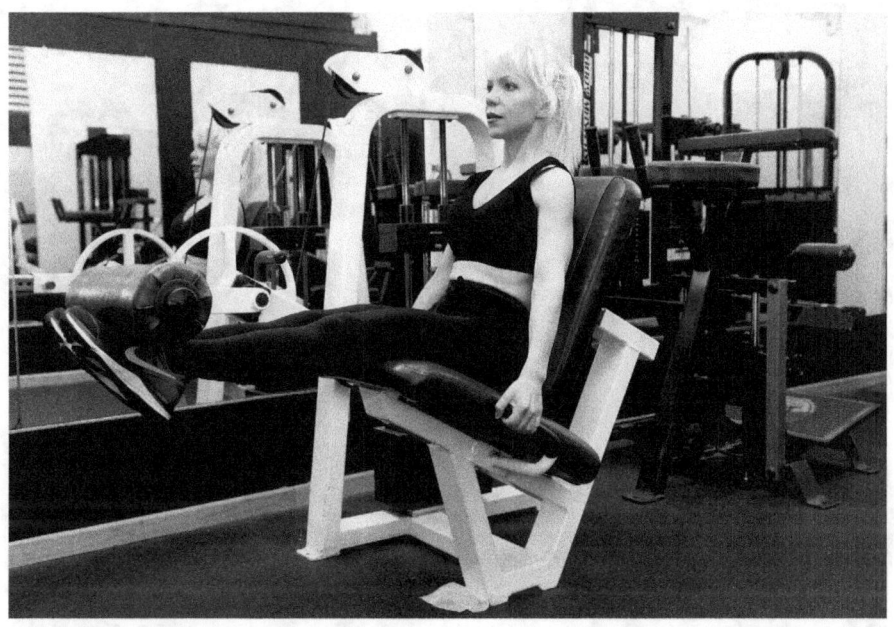

Breathe in, and then breathe out as you straighten the legs. Don't lock the knees in the straight position.

Breathe in as you return to the starting position.

Count to three as you straighten the legs, and count to three as you return to the starting position.

The image below shows incorrect form.

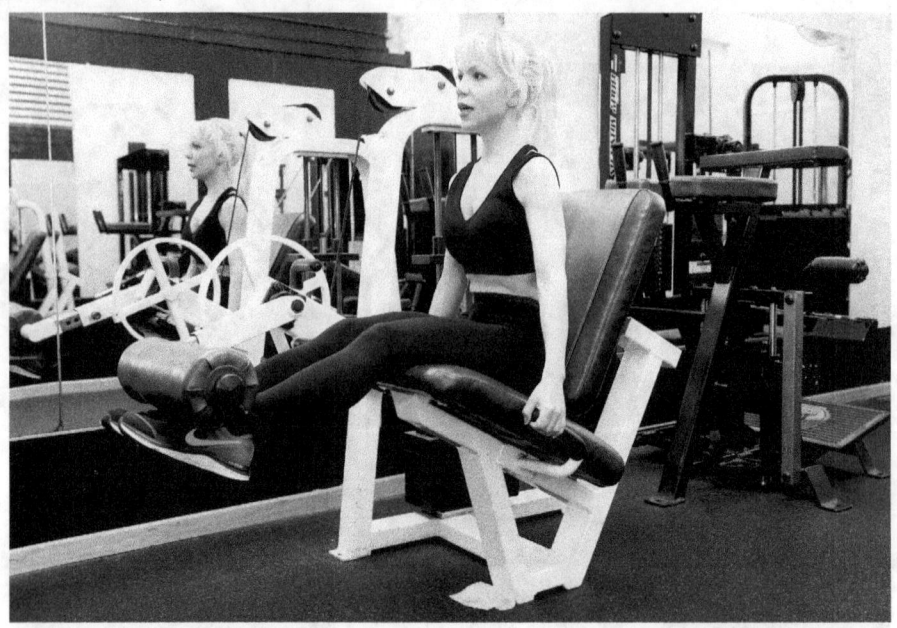

Here, the knees are not straight at the extension. Unless you have a knee injury and can't straighten the leg fully, this fails to develop the part of the quadriceps that holds the patella (knee cap) in place. If there is pain in the knee as you straighten the leg, lower the weights or extend the leg only as far as you can without pain.

Another common mistake is using momentum to lift the foot lever, or arching the back during the movement. Arching the back or "swinging" the upper body as you extend your legs strains the back. The shoulders should stay flat on the back pad during the movement.

8) THE HAMSTRINGS (BICEPS FEMORIS)

PRONE HAMSTRING CURLS

Three sets, 12 repetitions.

Rest 30 to 60 seconds between sets.

This machine needs to be adjusted to your height. On most machines, you can adjust the bottom lever, the one that rests on the calves. If adjusted correctly, it rests just above the heels.

The knees should not rest on the bottom part of the machine, but should stick out over the rim, so there's no pressure on the kneecap.

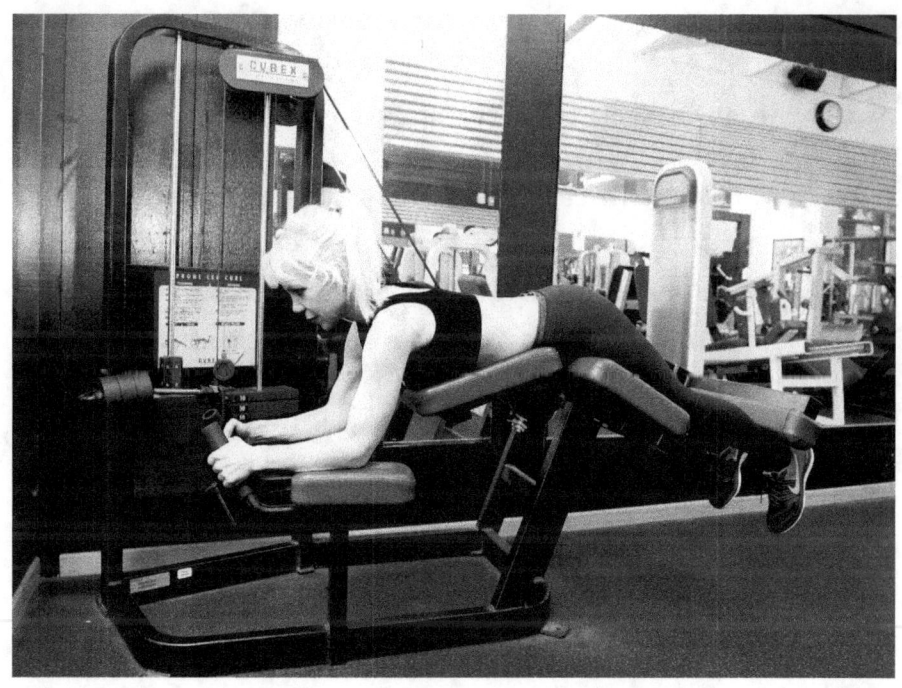

Lay prone on the machine, holding on to hand rails. Keep

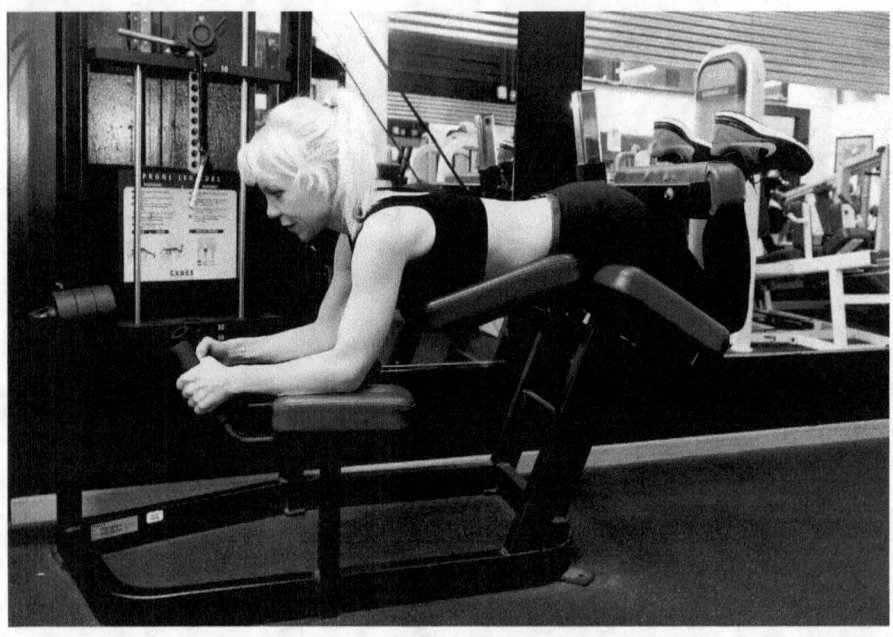

Breathe in, and then breathe out as you pull your heels toward your buttocks.

Breathe in as you return to the starting position.

Lower the lever with care. Don't lock the knees at the end of the movement, but maintain muscular tension and a slight bend. On most machines, you prevent the knees from locking by not allowing the weight stacks of the machine to touch.

Count to three as you bend the legs, and count to three as you return to the starting position.

The image below shows incorrect form.

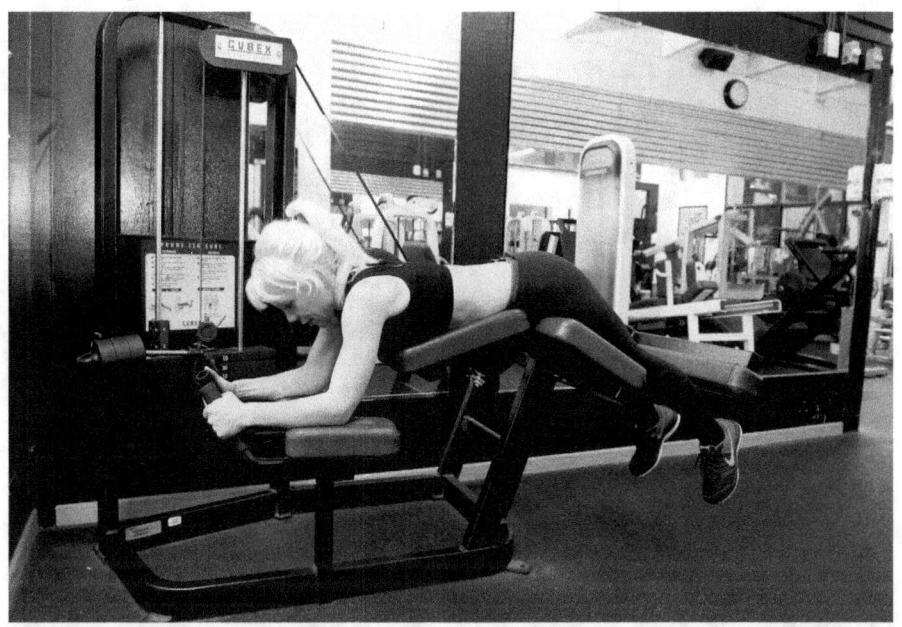

Here, you see the knees locked at the bottom of the exercise. The heels are not holding up the foot lever. This is appropriate during rest but not throughout the set as it doesn't optimize muscular tension. Additional common mistakes include using upper body momentum to lift the foot lever, or arching the back during the movement.

9) THE CALF (SOLEUS)

SEATED CALF RAISE

Three sets, 12 repetitions.

Rest 30 to 60 seconds between sets.

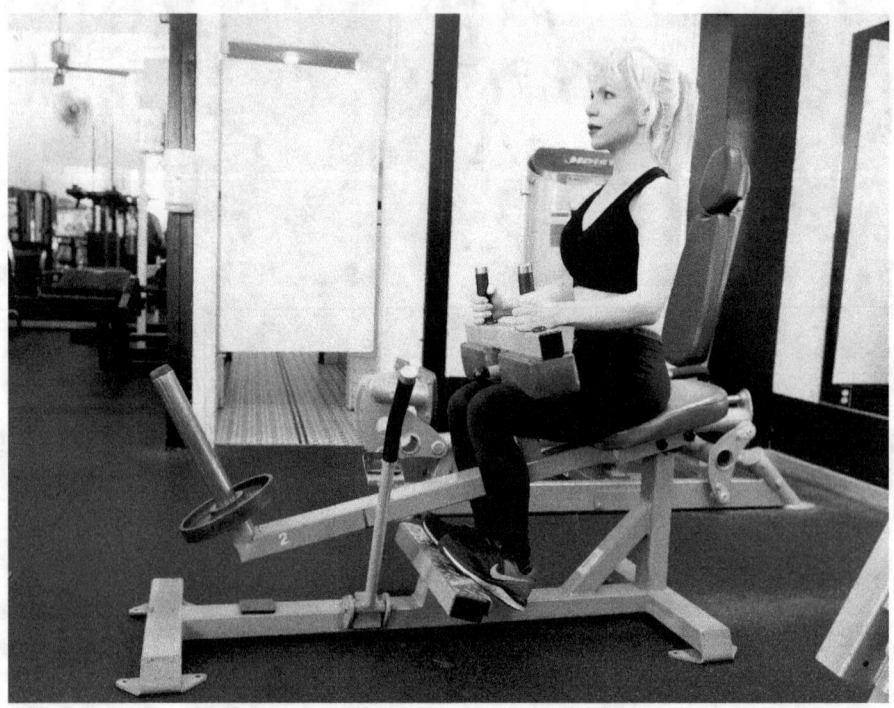

Start with your heel pointed down, so that you feel a stretch in your calf. The knees should be sticking out from underneath the knee pads, so there's no pressure on the knee.

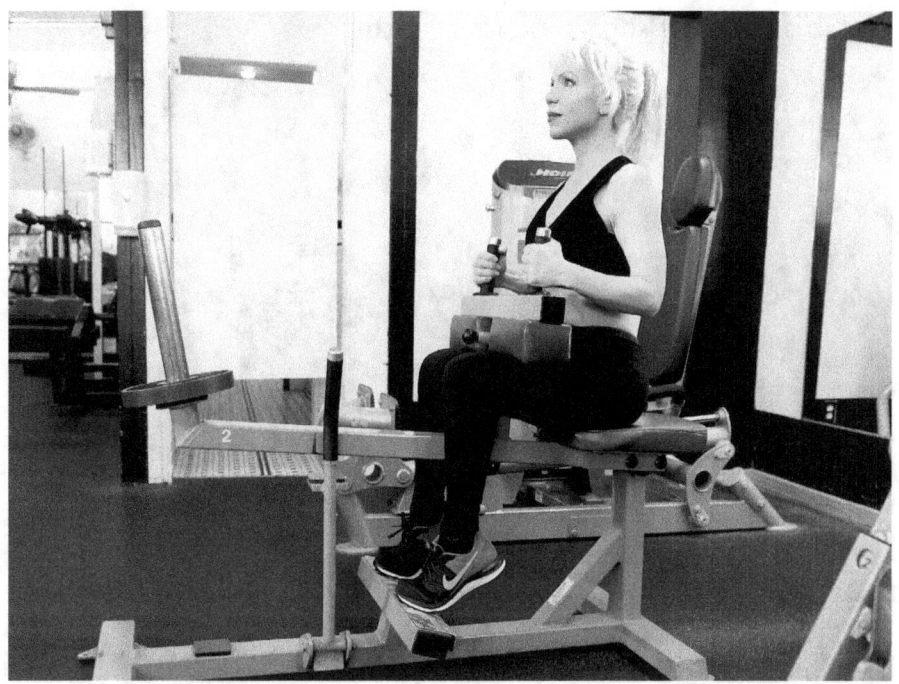

Breathe in, and then breathe out as you lift to the tips of your toes.

Breathe in as you return to the starting position.

Count to three as you lift, and count to three as you return to the starting position.

The image below shows incorrect form.

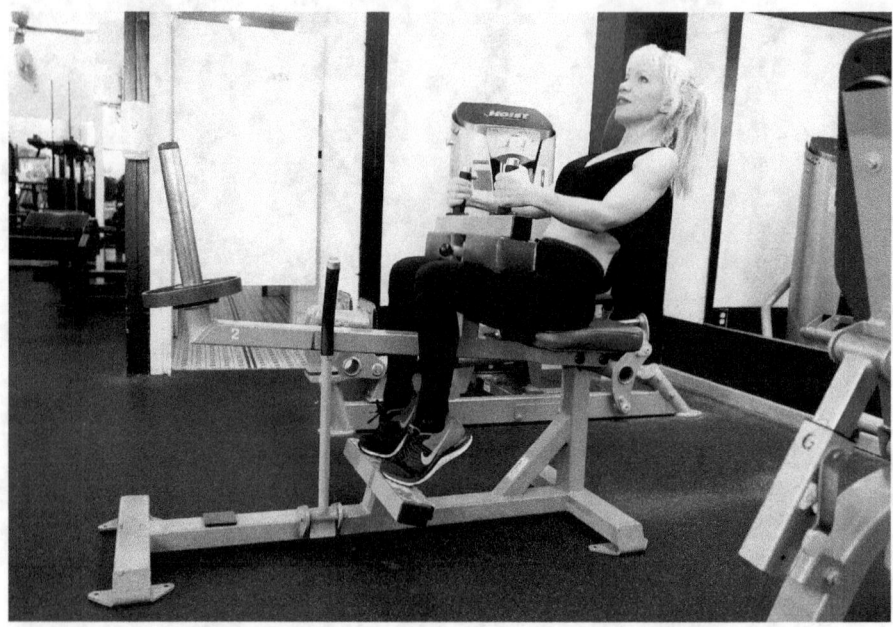

Here, the weight is moved by using upper body momentum and swaying backward. I'm exaggerating the movement so you can see the mistake. This fails to engage the muscle and may strain the back. Additional common mistakes include resting the machine lever on top of the knee, which creates pressure on the patella.

CHAPTER 2

STRETCHING

1) HAMSTRING STRETCH WITH RUBBER BAND

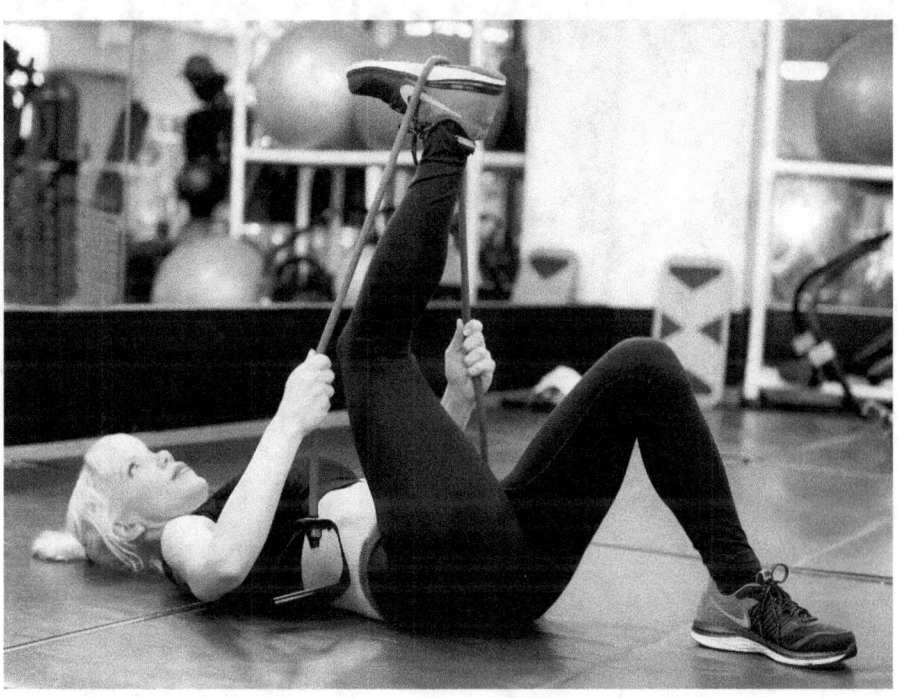

Lay on a mat, keeping your back straight and one knee bent. Wrap the rubber band securely around the foot of your other leg.

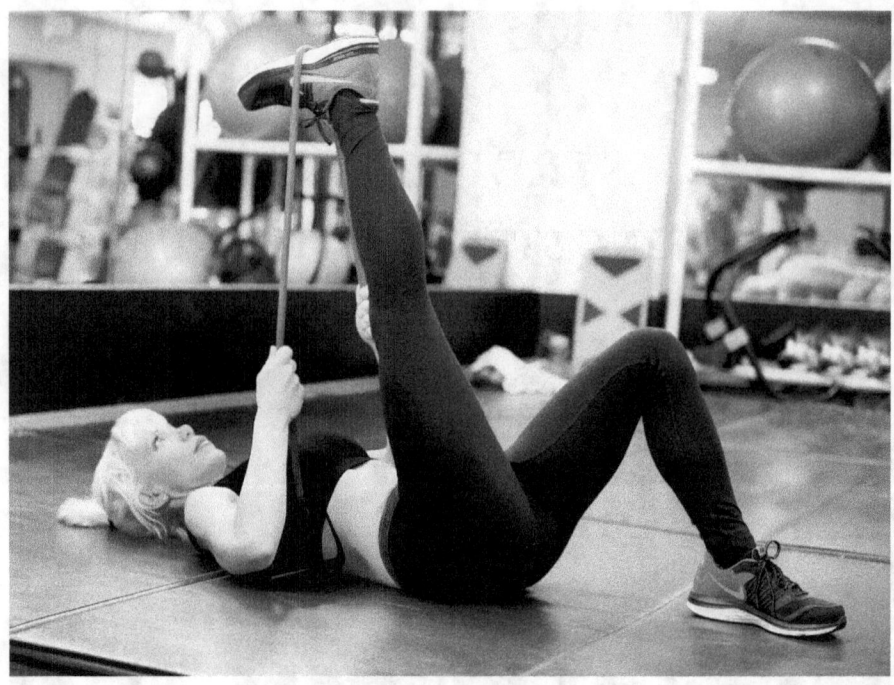

Slowly straighten the leg, pulling toward your chest.

Relax and allow the pulling sensation on the back of your leg. When you are properly warmed up, the pull won't hurt you. It will become more comfortable over time.

Don't allow your hips and buttocks to lift off the floor. Hold for 30 to 60 seconds. Repeat two to four times per leg.

2) LOWER BACK STRETCH

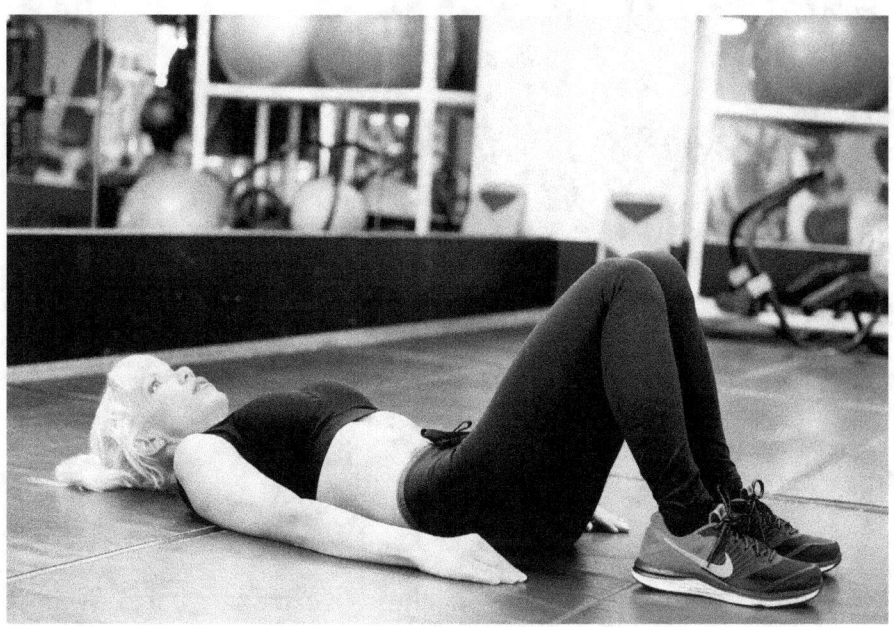

Lie on the mat with your knees bent.

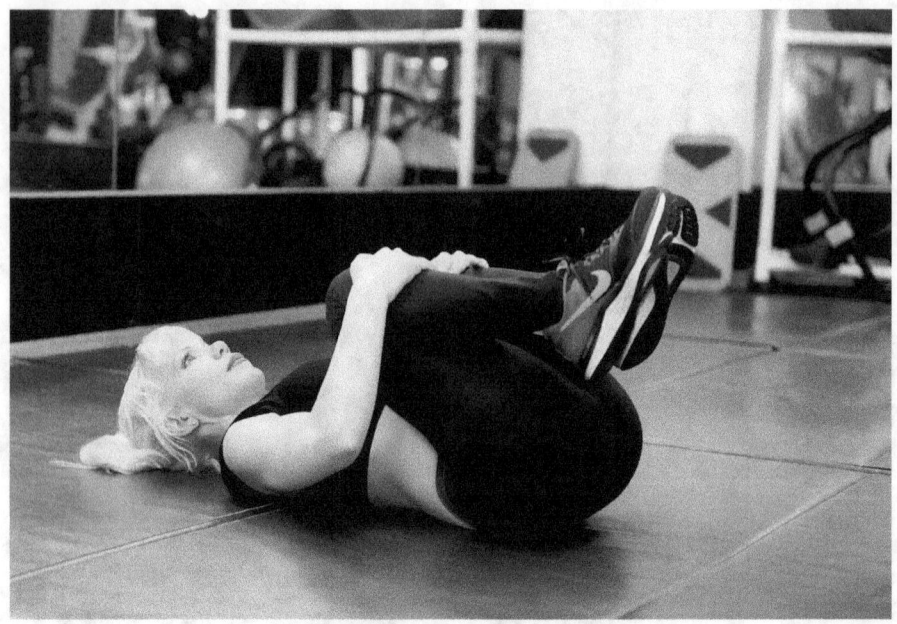

Hug your knees tightly to your chest. Keep your back straight and your hips down. It should feel as if you are using your bent legs to press the spine flat against the floor.

Allow the spinal stretch until the entire back is loose enough to touch the floor.

Hold for 60 seconds. Repeat two to four times.

3) MID-BACK STRETCH

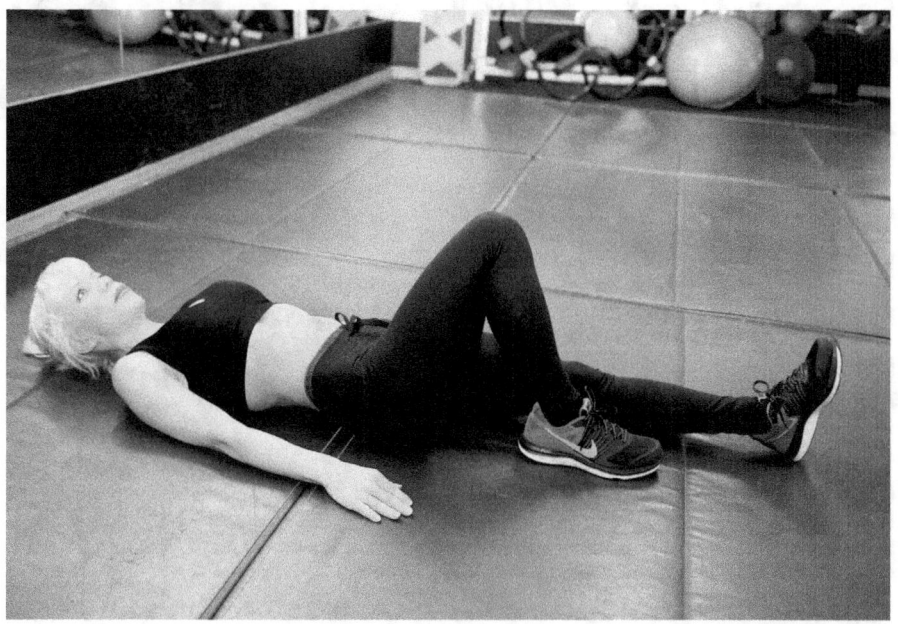

Lie on the mat, bend one knee and keep the other leg straight.

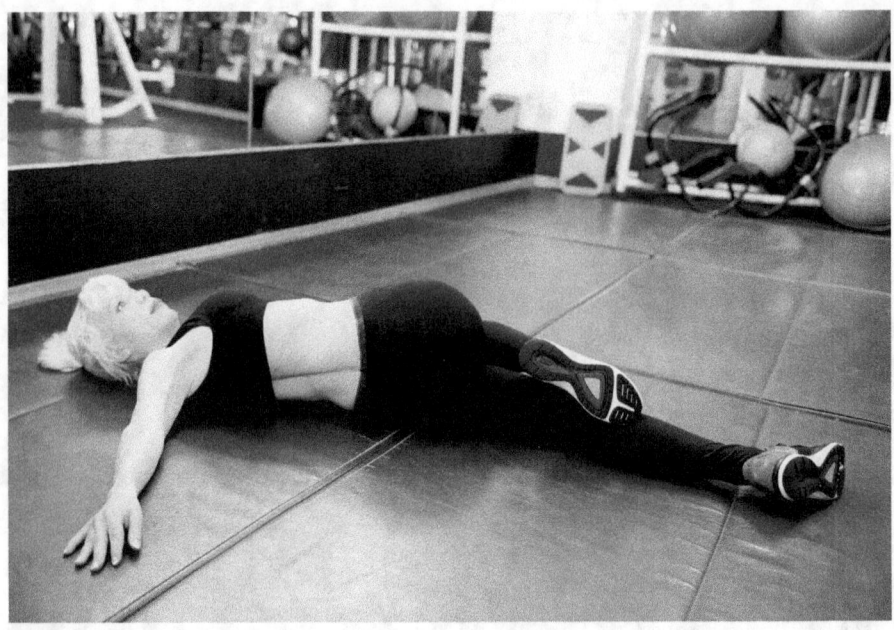

Bring the bent knee across the straight leg, pushing it gently toward the floor so it creates a "twist in the middle". Be mindful of keeping your shoulders flat on the floor. Keep upper body, pelvis and extended leg in a straight line.

Relax as your lower and mid-back loosen up.

Hold for 30 to 60 seconds. Repeat two to four times on both sides.

4) INNER THIGH STRETCH

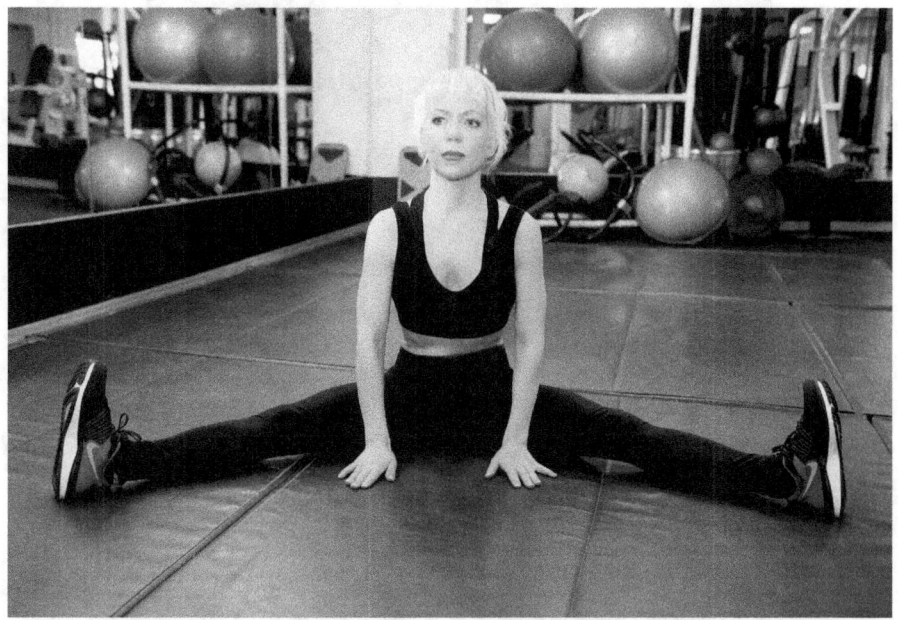

Sit on the mat with your back straight, legs in a V-position. If this position is uncomfortable in the beginning, start with a very small "V". Straighten the legs as much as you can. Be gentle with yourself. It will become easier over time.

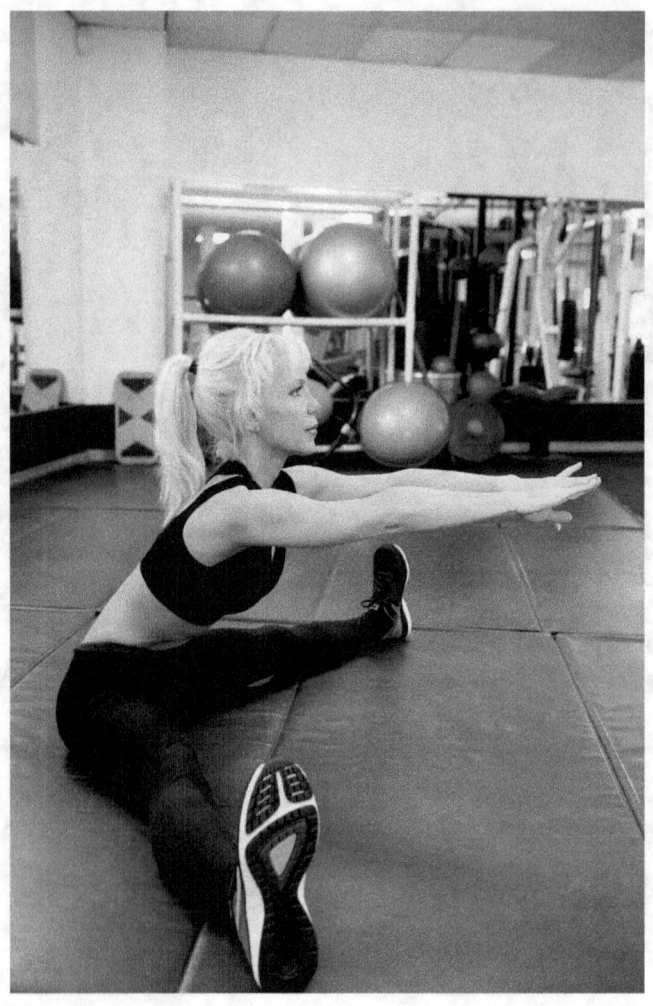

Gently pull the upper body forward. Extend the arms to help maintain a straight back.

Relax as you allow the stretching sensation in the inner thighs. Be mindful not to strain your lower back. If there is discomfort in the lower back, decrease the stretch and check that your back is straight.

Hold for 30 to 60 seconds. Repeat two to four times.

146

5) HIP FLEXOR STRETCH

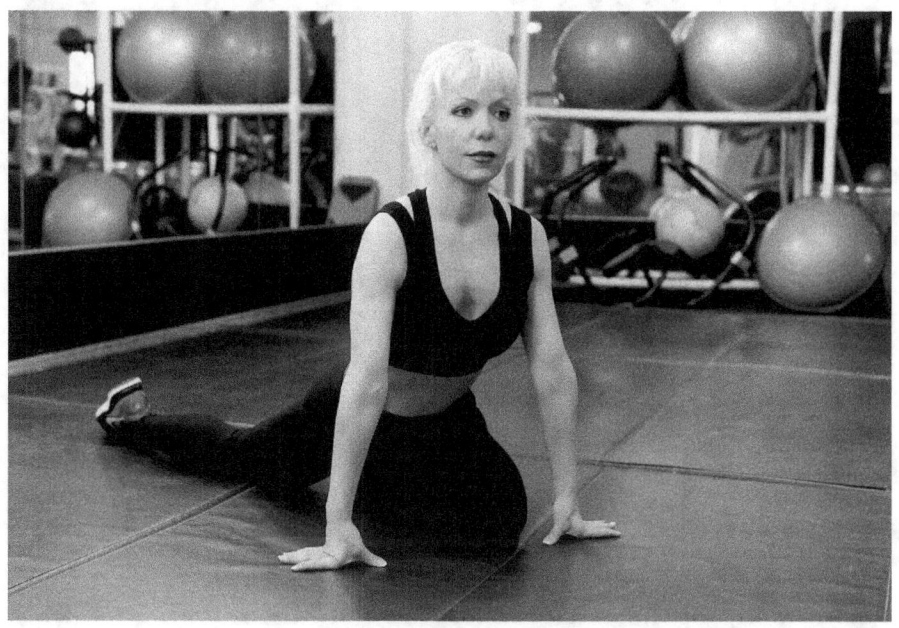

Sit on a bent leg, extending the other leg backward.

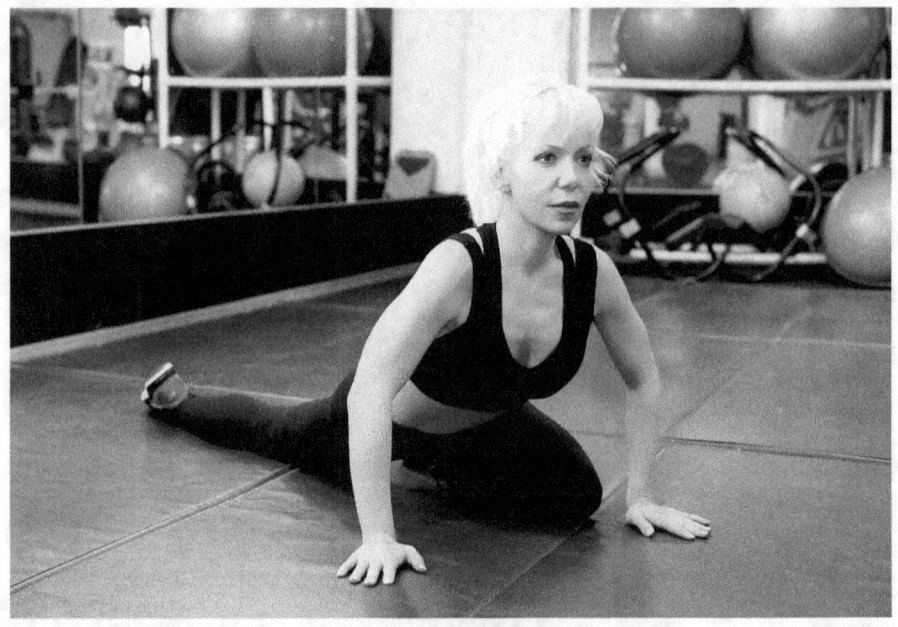

Push the hip of the extended leg gently to the floor.

Relax as you allow the pull in the hip on the side of the extended leg.

Hold for 30 to 60 seconds. Repeat two to four times on both sides.

PART 4:
CREATING BEAUTY:
ADVANCED EXERCISE
TECHNIQUES AND THE ART
OF BODYSCULPTING

Chapter 1

SET YOUR GOAL, ONE GOAL AT A TIME

Let's talk about goals. When discussing exercise, the best goal you can make is a simple one, such as completing a cycle of exercise.

What's the point in exercising if you don't have a goal to accomplish? Where's the motivation?

We're so conditioned to set and achieve goals that not working toward a goal seems counterproductive. But it isn't.

If you go through an intense bout of exercise because you're working toward being in the best shape of your life for a wedding or other life event, you may give yourself too little time, work too hard, too fast and do damage to your musculoskeletal frame. The novelty will wear off once you've achieved your goal.

What's next? A new goal will move into sight. You may refocus, quit exercising to gather energy and time for the new goal, and lose your gains.

A goal-orientation is not a good motivational foundation for fitness. Rather, relate to exercise and fitness as a lifestyle or a lifestyle change. You'll still have a goal, such as feeling better, loving your body and experiencing yourself as desirable. You'll still have an inherent goal in the cycle of exercise you're going through, such as building a foundation, sculpting or maintaining.

Relate to exercise and fitness as a process, not an event. A process is less goal-oriented and more intrinsically motivated, but it still progresses in stages and produces change. Intrinsic motivation is feeling better and loving your body. Extrinsic motivation is focusing on looking a certain way within a certain time span.

The stages of fitness are the cycles of training.

THE CYCLES OF TRAINING

The first cycle is changing body composition and building a solid foundation for your musculoskeletal frame. After building a foundation over three to nine months, you'll have enough lean muscle mass to move into the art of bodysculpting. This is where the real fun begins.

You can only appreciate the real fun of sculpting your body if you have enough lean muscle mass, which is your sculpting material. You can't rush it or cheat it, and there is no exact formula for how long it will take.

In the beginning cycle, you exercise the entire body and all the major muscle groups. You should notice a significant difference after a month of weightlifting three times per week. The beginning cycle doesn't have to be limited or boring; it's when you learn "exercise vocabulary" or the many different exercises for each muscle group. You begin with machines, move on to barbells, and eventually dumbbells. You'll learn combinations and circuits.

If you continue changing your body composition into more lean mass and less fat, lean strong lines will emerge where flab once resided. You will be intimately familiar with each muscle group, recognize the feeling of muscular fatigue or recovery, and experience increasing body awareness.

In the advanced cycles, sculpting muscle becomes easy when you're intimately familiar with growth and recovery. You've paid close attention to the various muscle groups and you've cared for their needs. By paying attention, listening, caring and tending to it, your body becomes your sculpture and your personal work of art. Shaping or sculpting will make a lot of sense, because you've learned how to grow muscle and you're familiar with the process of physical change.

Eventually, you'll look in the mirror and decide to make your waist a tad smaller, lift the buttocks an inch or so, decide on a leaner line of the inner thigh or sculpt a nicely rounded deltoid so the sleeve of a pretty blouse will bounce nicely off the muscle. This is the art of bodysculpting. Bodysculpting is the process of changing or altering shapes to your liking.

Bodysculpting is broken down into separate cycles.

Sculpting cycles are shorter than the beginning building cycle. Sculpting cycles may alter every month, depending on how ambitious you are. Some cycles may be dedicated to increasing the size of a muscle (making the back side of the upper arm harder, for example) whereas other cycles may be dedicated to increasing the definition of the muscle (making the back side of the arm a clean, clear line)

The process of bodysculpting requires more in-depth knowledge of manipulating the growth or shape of muscle groups. For now, I want to give you a basic understanding of what's ahead and how it's done. Let's discuss some advanced exercise techniques.

EXERCISE VARIETY

Advanced exercise is relative. When you're at the gym for the first time, every exercise is new. After you've mastered the Basic Workout, each new exercise is an advancement.

Let's start with the first increment of advancement, which is learning variety.

Depending on your knowledge of gym equipment, you can use various exercises. For example, if you know several exercises for the chest, you can alternate. You can use the chest press machine featured in the practical instruction section, or you can use any other exercise as long as you're sure it's targeting the same muscle group.

You can work all major muscle groups of the Basic Workout, but vary the exercises you choose.

When alternating exercises, be sure to maintain consistent intensity. Intensity is the number of sets and repetitions paired with the amount of weight you're lifting. If you're working the chest at a 7 on the Scale of Perceived Exertion, keep working at a 7 on any chest exercise. You can alternate the way you work a muscle, but don't alternate the stress you put on it.

No exercise is superior to another. Different exercises work different aspects of a muscle.

Exercise bands, machines, free weights or any new exercise gadget merely provides different stimulation to a muscle. The more "vocabulary" you have, the more creative you can be. There is no single exercise gadget that can give you a perfectly sculpted muscle. Perfect sculpture is the result of a perfect combination. Perfect combinations result from working a muscle's different aspects, which we'll discuss in another section.

Machines are safer and more suitable for beginners. Beginners need to learn the range of motion of each muscle group. In other words, you need to learn which way a limb is supposed to move naturally, and which way it's not supposed to move. When you use machines, the direction of movement is limited to what's safe. You learn the safe range by using machines, and you can then move on to free weights.

When using free weights, there is unlimited range of motion. The weights can go any way when you lift. You have to balance free weights carefully throughout a correct arch of motion. Don't do it until you know the correct arch.

Variety is a good thing for avoiding mental boredom and physical plateauing. Expand your "exercise vocabulary" as much as you can.

Limiting yourself to exercises you enjoy will give you limited results. Whether or not you like an exercise should not be a decisive factor. Do you want a physical frame that lasts? Do you want to actualize the magnificent beauty that dwells within your physical potential? Then don't think in terms of what you like. Think in terms of what needs to be done.

Once you have a good vocabulary of exercises, this is going to be easy. However, you can continue to use the same exercises for your first cycle if you want to keep it simple, because there is plenty of adaptation in the first three to six months.

ADVANCED TRAINING CYCLES

A training cycle should span across four to 12 weeks. During a training cycle, you can maintain the same exercises but increase intensity. The first cycle is the Basic Workout, and I heartily recommend allowing a minimum of 12 weeks before you move on to more advanced or strenuous routines.

Start with a 12-week cycle of three to four sets of 10 to 15 repetitions. Work your abdominals at a higher number of sets and repetitions, because there are no weights involved and the intensity is much lower.

You may start with 10 repetitions if you find it's all you can do comfortably. Stay with it for four to six weeks and move on to 12 to 15 repetitions in the second half of the cycle. You may start with three sets and move on to four sets once you feel stronger. Listen to your body during the workout and the day after, and adjust the intensity according to how your body responds. There is no "one size fits all" recipe to success. Make sure you worked enough to feel fatigued, but not to a point of pain.

Advanced cycles vary the number of sets and repetitions according to the purpose of the cycle.

The faster you exhaust a muscle, the more it grows. Sets of six repetitions grow larger muscle than sets of 15 repetitions. Definition is created by a mixture of growth (few repetitions) and burnout (high repetitions). Cycles of definition follow cycles of growth.

BUILDING DIFFERENT ASPECTS OF A MUSCLE

Let's make this a preview for things to come. You don't need advanced techniques during your first cycle, but it certainly doesn't hurt to know why your gym invested in all this clutter. Different exercises do slightly different things.

Any exercise focuses on a certain aspect of a muscle. It may be the middle, outer or inner portion, upper or lower portion. While the entire muscle group is involved on the job, the featured aspects get a bit more work done.

When you have a large exercise vocabulary, you'll know specific exercises that work certain muscle groups, as well as which aspect of the muscle is favored. When you do, you can work like an architect.

You can exercise the *outer chest* and build up the *lower, middle,* and *upper* "floor."

You can work the *inner chest* and build up *lower, middle,* and *upper* "floor."

For example, a chest press works the outer aspect of the chest muscle, and a chest fly works the inner aspect. While both machines will suffice to work the chest, the art of bodysculpting capitalizes on knowing which machine focuses on the desired aspect of a muscle. If you work only lower or upper floor, you'll still get stronger and improve your posture but you won't achieve the chiseled look of a sculpture.

When you're moving through advanced building and sculpting cycles, you will want to combine exercises skillfully, so you sculpt every muscle in its full glory. If you think you won't be interested, think again. Wouldn't you want to shape the buttocks so they're lifted above the line of the thighs, perky in the center as to defy gravity, and tight enough that they don't make the top of your thighs look like saddlebags? Yes, this can be done if you know how to combine exercises and work all aspects of a muscle.

As a general guideline, exercising with your arms closer to the spine works the inner aspect of an upper body muscle, and working with the arms farther away from the body's middle works the outer aspect.

Arms in = inner aspect of the muscle

Arms out = outer aspect of the muscle

The reverse is true for the legs. A stance that keeps the feet together works the outer part of the legs and buttocks. A wide stance works the inner thigh.

Feet close together = outer aspect of the muscle

Feet wide apart = inner aspect of the muscle

Skilled, advanced workouts are changed every time, meaning the muscle groups are worked by using different exercises for every workout. This is where knowing how to use a large variety of exercise equipment pays off. Changing the resistance by using different equipment prevents you from the plateau or stale period of Shock-Adaption-Staleness.

One more word on advanced workout routines. Remember the rule of respecting architecture? Every workout routine should train **core, chest, back, shoulder, triceps, biceps, quadriceps, hamstrings,** and **calf,** the major muscle groups. You can switch up the order as long as you give them all attention.

Any workout routine is only a variation of the Basic Workout.

MOTIVATING YOURSELF

What if you've read it all, you try to drum up motivation but can't, and you still find exercise dreadfully annoying? Well, you're not alone. It is annoying. So are a lot of things.

There are a blessed few among us who genuinely love exercising, and they do it because it is so much fun. Typically, they are in their twenties and they have so much energy that they don't know what to do with it. Might as well take it to the gym.

But most of us mere mortals, or those who are a little older, rarely exercise because it is so much fun. And they rarely have so much energy that they don't know what to do with it.

So let's say you're a fitness non-enthusiast. You know you would feel better if you exercised and you'd like to be fit, maybe even look a little tighter overall—but!

You don't like going to the gym. You abhor the idea of pumping heavy weights until you turn red in the face and sweat pours like a fountain, or running on the treadmill like a hamster on a wheel and never arriving at a destination.

The most common justification sounds something like this: "I'd like to exercise, but I don't like going to the gym. I prefer to exercise outside. I want this to be fun. I want to do this for recreation."

Honestly, if you exercise for recreation, you're either one of the blessed few who are true athletes at heart or it's time you get a life.

Exercising for fun is like brushing your teeth and going to the dentist for fun. Do you stand in front of the mirror at night and say to yourself: "I'm going to brush and floss and flush with fluoride because this is so much fun. I can't wait to do it. I love it! I've been looking forward to this all day. I do this for recreation!"

Seriously. If you do that, fine, but just know you are a bit unusual.

My guess is that you brush, floss, and flush because you know it's necessary. It's necessary if you want to keep your teeth clean and healthy. It's necessary because you want to maintain quality of life and take care of yourself.

Exercise is the same.

Fitness is not for fun. It's a serious matter. It's fine to expect exercise to be somewhat enjoyable, but if fun and recreation are your main expectations, you aren't likely to stay strong and mobile throughout your lifespan. You'll quit and wither away because the novelty will wear off. The definition of recreational fun changes over time.

Fitness is not about fun. It's not a hobby.

Your level of fitness relates closely to your overall level of health and well-being, your energy levels, and how you age. Fitness is about how much you want out of life and for how long. Do you want to live a long, healthy life but be wheelchair bound because your legs no longer have the strength to carry you? Do you want to spend the last decades of your life lying down because your back gave out on you?

It's investing in a metaphorical retirement fund so you won't be poor in old age. It's an investment in life quality through sustained mobility.

It's hideous to go to a gym where you're in close quarters with others who perform repetitive movements on gym equipment, haul around pieces of iron that are ironically called dumbbells, or huff and puff on treadmills. It gets boring after a while.

Remind yourself that you're not doing this for fun.

You're doing this to maintain the strength of your heart so that increased oxygen flow can energize your body and your brain. You're doing this so you'll still be walking in old age. You're doing it to have enough energy available to do what you need to do today. So you can enjoy your life, because if your body goes out on you, you'll enjoy your life a whole lot less. You are doing this so you can enjoy being in the body you have.

Remind yourself daily, and throw out the idea that fitness should be fun. It's a discipline. It's not a goal, it's a process. Do it whether you feel like it or not. You'll reap the rewards for a long time.

LAST WORDS

Generally, the exercises featured here for the major muscle groups are simple and safe.

Please be aware that if you have a diagnosed condition, if you are female past age 45 or male past age 55, or experience pain in the chest while you exercise, you should consult your physician and get clearance for exercise. Also, if you are past 60 years of age, you may want to consult a professional trainer for alternate abdominal exercises.

Enjoy your first cycle of exercise and congratulate yourself that you're on the way to bringing out the beauty and healthful functionality that has always been your potential.

I hope my take on fitness makes a difference in your life, and that my explanations made sense and were easy to understand without being too simplistic.

I'm 44 years old in the pictures. I had the occasional double chin or skin fold retouched, which couldn't be avoided when showing common mistakes, but I didn't retouch the body. What you see is a realistic physical goal for someone who is willing to exercise regularly and eat consciously. I'm not genetically lucky; I was overweight in my twenties and tried every diet until I found an approach to exercise that worked. I've been teaching this approach to clients for nearly two decades. If I wasn't exercising, I probably couldn't keep my weight, but I'd also be a regular at an orthopedic surgeon's office. I have arthritis in both knees and two herniated discs in the lumbar spine.

I hope you will be inspired to define the shape you want your body to be in, and have the necessary skills to create it. It can be done.

No matter how old you are, how much you weigh, or what your state of health is, you can get back into your body. There is no prescribed size for beauty or the sensual joy of physical expression. Listen to yourself only. Ignore external voices that tell you what shape your body should be in, unless it's your doctor's voice.

Listen closely, however. Body Dysmorphic Disorder and eating disorders will whisper in your ear that you are obese or grotesque looking and you need to lose weight when you don't. Obesity may whisper that you're just fine when you are not healthy.

Listen, and use good judgment about which inner voice is speaking to you. If you know your judgment is sound and you like the body you inhabit, reject external voices that demand your body should conform to someone else's standard. Enjoy your body; don't make it a battlefield.

And most of all, don't forget that you are *not* your body. You are more than just a body. Don't buy into the narcissistic hysteria of physical perfection. The body is the temple of your spirit or your true self. Make it a nice temple, but don't forget who you are.

If you enjoyed this book, please leave a review on Amazon.

Thank you!

If you want to be notified of upcoming titles or receive a free copy during promotions, please sign up to my mailing list at: _www.ViviStutz.com/contact.html_.

ABOUT THE AUTHOR

VIVI STUTZ writes both non-fiction and fiction. She is a Certified Personal Trainer and Orthopedic Exercise Specialist through the American Council on Exercise, and a pre-licensed Marriage and Family therapist with two Masters degrees in psychology and in spiritual psychology.

Originally from Germany and now a dual citizen, she lives in Southern California with her husband and a hoard of rescue animals.

www.ingramcontent.com/pod-product-compliance
Lightning Source LLC
Chambersburg PA
CBHW060106300526
45787CB00018B/317